Routine Outcome Monitoring and Feedback in Psychological Therapies

Routine Outcome Monitoring and Feedback in Psychological Therapies

Kim de Jong, Jaime Delgadillo and Michael Barkham

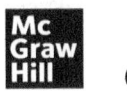 Open University Press

Open University Press
McGraw Hill
Unit 4
Foundation Park
Roxborough Way
Maidenhead
SL6 3UD

email: emea_uk_ireland@mheducation.com
world wide web: www.openup.co.uk

First edition published 2023

A catalogue record of this book is available from the British Library

ISBN-13: 978-0-3352-4969-5
ISBN-10: 0335249698
eISBN: 978-0-3352-4970-1

Library of Congress Cataloging-in-Publication Data
CIP data applied for

Typeset by Transforma Pvt. Ltd., Chennai, India

Praise page

"This is an outstanding book. The depth and breadth of these authors' knowledge about progress monitoring shine through on every page. The book provides an essential guide for clinicians and organizations who wish to use progress monitoring in their daily work. A large body of evidence shows that if you simply take the step of monitoring your clients' progress, they will have better treatment outcomes. What could be better than that?"
Jacqueline B. Persons, Director, Oakland Cognitive Behavior Therapy Center
and Clinical Professor, Department of Psychology,
University of California at Berkeley, USA

"Where can I sign up for the de Jong, Delgadillo, and Barkham fan club? Their book is clear, well-written, evidence-based, and timely. Combined with their decades of practice-based research and clinical experience, it describes a way helping professionals of all stripes can improve the results of psychological care."
Scott D. Miller, Ph.D., International Center for Clinical Excellence

"This is the first real practice book on Routine Outcome Monitoring (ROM) and feedback. It provides therapists with very concrete information on introducing measurement into treatment, interpreting the scores and discussing them with the patient. In addition, it is instructive for the manager who wants to implement ROM and the supervisor who uses ROM in supervision. The book is very clearly written with telling examples. Each chapter ends with the key points, which make it easy to retain the main points or refresh them later. Highly recommended for anyone working in the mental health field."
Prof. Dr. Bea Tiemens, Professor of Evidence-based practice
in mental health care at Radboud University, Nijmegen, NL.
Head of Research department in Pro Persona Mental Health Care,
Renkum, NL

"Today's practicing clinicians of the psychological therapies are faced with a major challenge - how to enhance clinical practice and interventions by implementing existing, easy to use and effective routine outcome monitoring into daily routine. This remarkable and hugely practice-oriented book helps clinicians not only with the knowledge and skills needed to tackle this task, but also elevates their abilities in using such systems. It covers the fundamental research concepts and offers practical training exercises to enhance treatment options and effectively use monitoring tools. With its extensive coverage and engaging style, this book is

sure to drive progress in the practice of psychological therapies around the world. I full heartedly endorse this book on routine outcome monitoring as a comprehensive and enjoyable read that will move the practice of psychological therapy forward."

Dr. Wolfgang Lutz, Department of Psychology,
University of Trier, Germany

"The authors graciously acknowledge the visionaries in the field who paved the way for feedback informed treatment and routine outcome monitoring (ROM), such as Kenneth Howard and Michael Lambert, but they really are true visionaries themselves. They have given us a book containing all you need to know about how to track progress in psychotherapy. I particularly liked the way the authors discuss not only the unquestionable advantages of ROM, but also the challenges and provide excellent advice how to overcome them and to create a culture of learning and feedback. This is a must-read for every therapist, supervisor, researcher, manager – and client – in the field of mental health."

Helene A. Nissen-Lie, Clinical Professor and Therapist,
University of Oslo, Norway

"I highly recommend this book to anyone wanting to work with a routine outcome monitoring (ROM) and feedback system in psychological therapies. It provides a review of relevant research, guidance on the challenging task of setting up ROM and describes ways of identifying and helping clients who are not improving. This book from three leading clinical researchers in the field is scholarly, practical and timely."

Professor Mike Lucock, Centre for Applied Research in Health,
University of Huddersfield, UK

To Michael J. Lambert, a beloved friend and esteemed colleague,
on whose shoulders we stand.

Contents

Foreword

We have seen many purported innovations in the field of psychotherapy. Every year brings a new treatment based on a new approach to a particular disorder, based on advances in basic psychological sciences, say in cognitive or neuro-psychology. Unfortunately, many of these innovations have been found to be no more effective than previous approaches. Some of these innovations are interesting, but bring us no closer to the goal of quality improvement in clinical practice.

Despite the disappointing results of some developments in the field, one innovation has consistently demonstrated its utility. Routine outcome monitoring (ROM, also referred to as practice-based evidence, feedback informed treatment, measurement-based care) is defined as using information about patient progress and the process of therapy, collected regularly, to guide therapy. First proposed by Ken Howard and developed by Michael Lambert, Len Bickman, and Michael Barkham, among others, ROM has been rigorously examined in randomized clinical trials, and meta-analyses have consistently shown that the use of ROM improves outcomes. ROM is a transtheoretical practice that improves outcomes—that is, regardless of the theoretical approach used, ROM will result in better outcomes.

Despite the strong evidence for ROM, implementation in practice is not straightforward. There are a variety of measures and systems, methods for determining satisfactory progress, and ways to present the information to therapists. Research shows that adequate implementation of ROM is critical to its success. As is the case with any practice, there are best practices that optimize outcomes. Unfortunately, most of what is known about ROM exists in the scientific literature but it is not easily accessible to clinical services and practitioners.

ROM is being widely adopted around the world, and in many systems ROM is a standard of care, either mandated or recommended in practice guidelines. What is urgently needed is a resource for clinicians and managers of care. Kim de Jong, Jaime Delgadillo, and Michael Barkham are three of the premier ROM researchers—and they have extensive experience of implementing ROM in large systems of care. The authors are also very active members in international research organizations and conferences focusing on ROM, such as the Society of Psychotherapy Research (SPR). This is the ideal background to author *Routine Outcome Monitoring and Feedback in Psychological Therapies*, which will be the seminal source that clinicians and managers will use as they implement and utilize ROM.

As a "practitioner's guide", the book reaches out to therapists, who have lacked access to the resources and practical guidelines to implement ROM. Furthermore, the book also provides scientific background information, while maintaining a practical and implementation-oriented focus. The book's main readership are psychological and mental health professionals who are either interested in incorporating routine outcome monitoring and feedback systems into their clinical work or who are faced with challenges as they implement such systems at an institutional or service level. As such, the book is a suitable resource for clinical training and continued education courses for beginners as well as experienced clinicians. As the implementation of such systems increases in health care organizations, a growing number of clinical training programs are using and teaching ROM and feedback, and this book will be an important resource for mental health trainees. Practicing clinicians, facing multiple challenges, will find the book a straightforward, clear and concise guide for implementing ROM in their practice.

One of the many strengths of this book is the independent and unbiased survey of available measures and feedback systems without conflicts of interest associated with a commercial interest in or allegiance to a specific feedback system. This way, practitioners are provided a comprehensive overview of what is available so they can make informed decisions that are appropriate for their setting, context and resources.

Wolfgang Lutz, Trier Germany

Bruce E. Wampold, Madison, Wisconsin, USA

Preface

Personal note from the authors

If you picked up this book, you are probably considering starting to use routine outcome monitoring (ROM), or maybe you are already using it and you are looking for guidance on how to make the most of it for your practice and your patients. Perhaps you have encountered challenges to implementing ROM in your team, or you are wondering how to fully integrate it into therapy sessions and clinical supervision processes. Or maybe you are undecided and unsure if ROM and feedback is something worth using. In all of these situations, we hope that this book will provide you with support and guidance on this topic.

There are many reasons to take interest in the use of ROM and feedback in psychological care. Current scientific evidence shows that it can improve treatment outcomes, reduce treatment dropout and improve the efficiency of psychological services. With the increased demand for mental health care, and limited resources to provide it, it is important to adopt innovations that help to improve the quality and effectiveness of psychological care. However, ROM is not yet a mainstream feature of psychological care across public and private treatment providers, nor is it a standard feature of mainstream psychotherapy training programmes. In our view, one of reasons for this is that psychological services and higher education institutions often do not know how to effectively implement ROM, and therapists do not always know how to effectively integrate it into their practice and supervision. This science–practice gap motivated us to write this book, with the aspiration to mainstream the use of ROM and feedback as an integral part of psychological treatment.

The content of this book is based on the latest research and theory in the field, on our own experiences of implementing ROM in a variety of mental healthcare settings, and our experience of using ROM and feedback as therapists and supervisors. One of the things that I (KdJ) love when using ROM in therapy, is when we discuss the ROM and a patient realizes the progress they have made since the start of treatment. I remember one of my first patients having a slight worsening of their depression after an initial improvement. It felt to them like they had made no progress at all and were back to square one. Showing the ROM graph was so helpful. It helped them to remember the progress they had made earlier. And that bump in the road did not mean that they had not already travelled some distance.

Personally, I could not imagine doing therapy without ROM, as it also helps me to signal when patients are not making sufficient progress and stimulates me to push myself and be creative with these patients. However, I jumped on the ROM train early in my career (during my master's degree), and am aware that not everyone may come to ROM with the same initial enthusiasm. And, of course, there have been examples in which ROM has been implemented poorly, causing it to be a burden to therapists and patients. Or situations in which ROM data was aggregated and used for political purposes, making it feel suspicious and unsafe. However, in our experience, when ROM is used in the way that it was intended, almost all therapists that we have trained and worked with like it, and patients especially appreciate it as part of treatment.

When we were writing this book, it was important to us that we wrote it independently of the many available outcome measures and ROM systems. The few practical books on ROM and feedback that have been published typically focus on one specific ROM system. In contrast, we have focused on the principles and processes of ROM, believing that it can be achieved with any (good enough) outcome measure. Of course, we do provide some guidance on how to choose potential measures. New ROM systems are being developed as we write, and while these may approach the measurement of treatment outcomes in a different way (e.g., using computerized adaptive testing) and may provide a different type of feedback (e.g., using symptom network models), the basic principles of how to work with this information in therapy will remain the same. Equally important to us was our wish to make the book applied – that is, practical. We specifically wanted it to be a book that would help therapists. When we are learning new therapy skills ourselves, what we appreciate most are examples from real patients and ideas of how to talk about these things with patients. This is why we included many examples of therapy dialogue and case vignettes in the book.

We recognize that we are, to some extent, limited by our own experiences, our own perspectives and our own approach in using ROM and feedback, primarily in the context of Dutch and English healthcare systems. This motivated us to include quotes throughout the book from patients, therapists working in different settings than ours, and researchers working in other countries. To achieve this, we have interviewed several prominent researchers who have studied ROM and feedback, as well as experienced clinicians who use ROM and feedback in their daily practice. We have also used information from interviews with patients and therapists that we collected (with appropriate permissions) in an earlier study (Delgadillo et al., 2017). Segments from the interviews are integrated throughout the book. In this way, the book pools the collective wisdom of many researchers, therapists and patients into a resource that can be of relevance to psychological services and clinical training programmes around the world.

Terminology used throughout the book

As we started writing this book, we recognized the importance of the language used to describe therapists, patients, and treatment settings. Different therapeutic orientations have different preferences in terminology. For therapists, the terms clinician and practitioner are also commonly used. While we use the expression *therapist* in this book, the terms can be used interchangeably. People seeking psychological therapy may be referred to as patients, clients, or service users. Humanistic and experiential therapists often prefer to use the term client. Policy documents, especially in the UK, usually apply the term service users. We favour the term *patient*, as research suggests that people seeking psychological treatment typically prefer this term (Mcguire-Snieckus et al., 2003; Simmons et al., 2010). We acknowledge that this may differ between settings and people have different preferences. When referring to a patient's gender, we have used the neutral pronoun *they*, with the exception of specific examples in quotes and boxes in which the patient's preferred pronouns were known. There are several places in the book where we refer to the UK Improving Access to Psychological Therapies (IAPT) programme. As of January 2023, IAPT has been renamed as 'NHS Talking Therapies for Anxiety and Depression'. However, for familiarity, we have retained the term IAPT in the text.

Reading guide

In writing this book, we aim to provide therapists with practical information on how to work with progress feedback in order to help to improve outcomes for patients in an easy and quick-to-read format, with many practical examples. Each chapter is organized in a standard way. It starts with a brief overview of the content in the section titled "In this chapter". In addition, each chapter (except Chapter 10), ends with a "Conclusions" and "Key points in this chapter" section, that summarize the main learning points of the chapter. In addition, the book is organized into three sections, and a final chapter that can be read independently. Hence, readers can determine where they want to enter the book depending on their own level of experience with ROM.

The first section of the book, comprising Chapters 1 and 2, provides the *academic underpinnings* of ROM and feedback. Chapter 1 discusses the history of outcome measurement, types of ROM as well as the scientific background for ROM and data–informed clinical decision making. Chapter 2 covers the principles for selecting ROM and feedback tools in clinical practice and provides an overview of procedures for implementing feedback instruments. Readers can start with this section or proceed straight to the later practical sections.

The second section, which includes Chapters 3 and 4, focuses on the *implementation* of ROM in services and in clinical practice. Chapter 3 discusses challenges for implementation and Chapter 4 provides recommendations and best practices for successful implementation of ROM. This section is most relevant to therapists with private (group) practices or managers of healthcare organizations who want to implement ROM and feedback in their services.

The third section is the most *applied section*, with practical examples, verbatim conversations with patients, and many illustrations of ROM and feedback graphs. It comprises Chapters 5 to 9 and details how therapists can work with ROM and feedback to enhance their patients' outcomes. Chapter 5 presents suggestions for clinicians about how to introduce ROM to patients and to support patient adherence. Chapter 6 helps practitioners to interpret scores as well as results from feedback systems. Chapters 7 and 8 discuss methods within ROM to identify cases that are not-on-track and to make the best use of ROM data to help those patients to benefit from therapy. Chapter 9 provides recommendations about the integration of ROM into clinical supervision and to establish an outcome-oriented supervision model.

Chapter 10, the final chapter, summarizes the knowledge synthesized in all previous sections and focuses on *consolidating* ROM and clinical feedback in psychological therapies to achieve a data-informed clinical practice.

Acknowledgements

When writing on the topic of ROM and feedback, it is fitting to thank those researchers who had the vision to develop ROM as an integral method in clinical practice. Kenneth I. Howard was one of those visionaries, who recognized a need to track patients' progress during treatment on a session-by-session basis. Michael J. Lambert, who developed one of the first ROM systems and conducted the first study of ROM and feedback, played a pivotal role in the development of this literature and has been a great friend, mentor and colleague to us. Similarly, Wolfgang Lutz, developer of one of the most sophisticated ROM and feedback systems, has truly revolutionized the field, and is a great friend and colleague to us all. In addition, we would also like to thank all the people who made time to be interviewed by us for the book: Robbie Babins-Wagner, Heidi Brattland, Susan Douglas, Hidde Kuiper, Wolfgang Lutz, John Mellor-Clark, Scott D. Miller, Christian Moltu, Andrew Page, Erik van der Put, and Terje Tilden. Thank you for sharing your wisdom and experiences, it has made the book so much richer and it was such a pleasure to have these conversations with each of you.

We would also like to thank Beth Summers and Hannah Jones at Open University Press for their faith in the process, their help and support, and their patience with us during the writing of the book during a global pandemic. Our thanks also to Joanna Priddy and Hidde Kuiper for giving feedback on drafts of a chapter, and Bea Tiemens and an anonymous reviewer for reading the first draft of the book and providing us with valuable feedback to help improve the book. Finally, Kim de Jong would like to thank her research assistants, who have been of great help with the administrative parts of getting the book together: Kanzi Hesham El Nasharty, Samia El Ulabi, and Vasiliki Kapetanou. Finally, we would like to thank our respective family members, who put up with us spending many evenings and weekends outside of our already long office hours working on the book.

Kim de Jong, Leiden, the Netherlands
Jaime Delgadillo, Sheffield, UK
Michael Barkham, Sheffield, UK

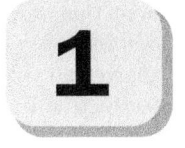

1

What is Routine Outcome Monitoring and why should I use it?

In this chapter

In this chapter, we provide you with a definition of what Routine Outcome Monitoring (ROM) entails and what the different goals of ROM are. We will start with a brief history of outcome assessment, then discuss the different types of ROM, including the combination of ROM and progress feedback. Next, we will discuss why therapists need systematic information on their patients' progress to aid clinical decision-making. Finally, we will review the evidence on the effectiveness of ROM and feedback in enhancing treatment outcomes from the scientific literature.

A brief history of outcome assessment

Early outcome assessment

Outcome assessment has a long history in the field of psychology (e.g., Codman, 1918). Since the early days of the profession, therapists have posited that psychotherapy can result in psychological and behavioural changes that can have a profound impact on the wellbeing of patients. These outcomes of therapy, however, are not always easily observable or evident. Behavioural outcomes, such as the frequency of an action (e.g., substance use) are possible to observe, measure and quantify. However, many other clinically relevant outcomes, such as emotional distress, are not so easy to evidence.

The first generation of outcome assessment in psychological interventions took place in the 1950s and 1960s and focused primarily on whether psychological interventions could change the personality of patients. During this period, outcome assessment comprised judgements by patients' own therapists, not based on any commonly used factor, but rather on so-called *impressionistic conclusions* (Lambert, 1983). At the time, the psychological treatment of choice was psychoanalysis, and there was a strong emphasis on the uniqueness of each patient. In 1941, Knight proposed to assess all patients on five 'reasonable criteria for measuring the success of an analysis' (p. 434), namely symptomatic recovery, increased productiveness, improved adjustment to and pleasures in the patient's sexual life, improved interpersonal relationships, and an improved ability to deal with psychological conflicts and stresses. The combined assessment of these five domains would result in a classification of treatment that was 'apparently cured', 'much improved', 'improved', or 'no change or worse'.

The second generation of outcome researchers focused on answering the question: which specific interventions and techniques are most effective for which specific disorders? Research from this period had limited generalizability, since many of these studies involved undergraduate students receiving therapy from trainee therapists. However, in this period, the use of standardized measures that were psychometrically sound became established. By *standardized measures* we refer to psychometric interview schedules or questionnaires that have a standard set of items, administration and scoring procedures, which have been validated for the measurement of clinically-relevant constructs (e.g., psychological problems, symptoms, processes, etc.).

The increasing political and economic pressure to demonstrate the effectiveness of psychological interventions eventually led to the third generation of outcome research (Drozd & Goldfried, 1996), in which there was a focus on using rigorous research methods. During this time period, randomized controlled trials (RCTs) were introduced in the field of psychology. Also during this time, the field of psychometrics had advanced considerably, and methods to design and to evaluate the validity and reliability of interviews and self-rated questionnaires had been established.

A higher degree of methodological rigour also introduced a higher degree of criticism from therapists on the usefulness of scientific research for their own practice. Therapists were unsure about what a statistical difference between two interventions meant and what the clinical implications of these results were for their own patients, who often did not resemble the patients included in the RCTs conducted at that time. This critique from therapists resulted in a series of articles in the late 1980s and early 1990s in which there was extensive debate on how to bridge the gap between science and practice (e.g., Clement, 1996; Drozd & Goldfried, 1996; Rainer, 1996). One consequence of this debate was the development of more intuitive and meaningful ways to define clinical outcomes, such as the concepts of clinical significance and reliable change (Jacobson & Truax, 1991).

Patient-focused research

As a consequence of developments in the field of psychometrics, and of the debate on bridging the gap between science and practice, a new research paradigm emerged with a focus on studying the treatments delivered in routine clinical practice. This line of research was introduced in the late 1990s and has been referred to as *practice-based evidence* (Barkham et al., 2001; Howard et al., 1996; Lambert et al., 2001) and *patient-focused research* (Lutz et al., 2015). It is based on the collaboration between therapists and researchers, in which therapists provide interventions and collect data by assessing their patients' progress using validated measures, and researchers analyse this information to study how therapy works in routine care (Lutz et al., 2015).

To gain a better understanding of patterns of change during the course of psychotherapy, it was vital that outcomes could be assessed more frequently, which led to the development of brief outcome measures that could be collected on a regular basis (e.g., Howard et al., 1996; Kadera et al., 1996). The traditional instruments to assess outcomes were too long to be used on a session-by-session basis and were often expensive due to license fees. In addition, developments in information technology systems and software packages enabled the development of computerized outcome monitoring charts and feedback systems. This enabled therapists to monitor their patients' progress during the course of treatment (Lutz, Deisenhofer et al., 2022).

Routine outcome monitoring

Routine outcome monitoring emerged as a consequence of some of the above historical developments. It has been described under various names, including *routine outcome measurement* (e.g., Bewick et al., 2006), *routine outcome monitoring, progress monitoring* (e.g., Byrne et al., 2012), *feedback informed treatment* (e.g., Delgadillo et al., 2018), *routine outcome monitoring feedback* (e.g., De Jong, 2016), *measurement feedback systems* (e.g., Bickman, 2008), *measurement-based care* (e.g., Scott & Lewis, 2015), *real-time monitoring* (e.g., Schiepek et al., 2016), and *outcome feedback* (e.g., Delgadillo et al., 2017).

Since its introduction, outcome monitoring and feedback have been implemented in a wide variety of mental healthcare settings worldwide, ranging from college counselling centres (e.g., Nordberg et al., 2018) to community mental health care (e.g., Connolly Gibbons et al., 2015), and from primary care settings (e.g., Delgadillo et al., 2017) to intensive inpatient treatment (e.g., De Jong et al., 2018) and emergency care inpatient settings (e.g., Van Oenen et al., 2016). It has also been applied to a wide variety of problems, including common mental health disorders, personality disorders, substance dependence, eating disorders, somatoform disorders, dissociative identity disorder, and psychotic disorders (e.g., Crits-Christoph et al., 2012; Davidsen et al., 2017; de Jong et al., 2018; Probst et al., 2013; Schiepek et al., 2016).

The American Psychological Association (APA) recommends the use of ROM and feedback methods in routine care (American Psychological Association, 2006), and the American Substance Abuse and Mental Health Services Administration (SAMHSA) has recognized two of the major feedback systems – the Outcome Questionnaire System (Lambert et al., 2004) and the Partners for Change Outcome Monitoring System (PCOMS; Miller et al., 2005) – as evidence-based interventions. The Joint Commission, an American accreditation organization, began requiring primary care and behavioural health providers who are treating mental health and substance use disorders to use standardized measures to inform treatment progress (Joint Commission, 2011). Similarly, the European research initiative ROAMER stated that there is a clear need for routine outcome monitoring as an accountability method to assess the effectiveness of treatments, therapists, and treatment centres (Emmelkamp et al., 2014). In addition, outcome monitoring is a key component of the Improving Access to Psychological Therapies (IAPT)[1] system in England (Clark, 2018). In many European countries, measuring treatment outcomes has been promoted, most prominently in the UK, Scandinavian countries, the Netherlands, and Germany. Australia was among the early adopters of outcome monitoring, and more recently, Asian countries such as China, Japan, and Taiwan have also introduced outcome monitoring in their mental health care systems.

What is Routine Outcome monitoring?

Definition and goals

In the literature, the term ROM has been used to signify different forms of measuring outcomes in routine care. Below, three different types of applications of outcome measures are described and Figure 1.1. summarizes the difference between them.

- *Routine Outcome Measurement*. This method typically involves measuring clinically relevant indicators (e.g., symptom severity, functioning, quality of life, etc.) at the start and end of treatment. Sometimes, additional measurements during therapy will be administered, but this method is characterized by low-frequency measurements that are conducted with the aim of evaluating a service's overall outcomes. Mental health care is costly, and to justify such an expenditure, organizations financing care (e.g., the government or insurance companies) may require evidence of its effectiveness. In addition, patients may want to know about the effectiveness of services or therapists when making decisions about seeking treatment or continuing a treatment that they are already accessing. In some countries this type of ROM contributes to the development of performance benchmarks, using data from different services to estimate and to compare their effectiveness. Such large-scale evaluations can help to understand the features of highly performing and underperforming services, which in turn can help to generate recommendations for the improvement of routine care (e.g., see Gyani et al., 2013). In this book, we will refer to this type of application as *outcome measurement*.
- *Routine Outcome Monitoring*. This method involves measuring clinically relevant indicators at frequent intervals during the course of treatment. It is characterized by high frequency measurements, such as on a session-by-session basis, or at less frequent fixed intervals (e.g., after every X number of sessions). Monitoring can be used for multiple purposes. In some settings the measures are used primarily for research purposes and accountability towards third parties, but in most settings, there is an explicit aim to use the measurements to inform treatment and aid clinical decision-making. In this book, when we use the term ROM, we refer to this type of application.
- *ROM and Feedback*. When outcome monitoring is supplemented with active messages to the therapist and/or patient that aid clinical decision-making, we refer to it as feedback. Without feedback, it can be difficult to decide whether a change in symptoms or functioning is clinically relevant,

or just a natural fluctuation or measurement error. Feedback enables therapists to make an informed decision about treatment progress. More advanced
feedback systems use statistical prediction models to compare a patient's
treatment progress against data from previous patients. Some computerized
systems can provide an automated signal to the therapist (and/or patient) to
alert them to cases where treatment is not working as well as expected.
These automated feedback signals can help therapists to investigate what
might be getting in the way of improvement and to make adaptations to
treatment. In this book, we will use the expression *ROM and feedback* when
we refer to this type of application.

A simple way to distinguish these three types of applications and concepts is
summarized in Figure 1.1. *Measurement* helps to obtain information about the
effectiveness of treatment. *Monitoring* helps therapists to track changes in
clinically relevant indicators and to inform their treatment plan and decisions.
ROM and Feedback helps therapists to become immediately aware of situations
when treatment is not working as well as expected, prompting them to identify
and deal with relevant problems. The main focus of this book is on *ROM and
feedback*.

Figure 1.1 Different applications of outcome measures

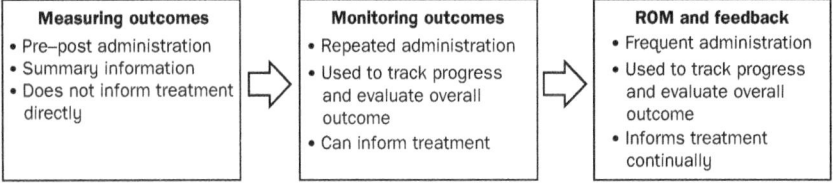

Different types of feedback

Broadly, there are three different types of progress feedback: feedback using
raw scores, feedback using expected treatment response (ETR) curves, and
feedback using a combination of ETR and clinical support tools (CSTs). All
feedback systems can help to alert the therapist when treatment is not progressing well. These situations are referred to as *not-on-track* cases (NOT) or
signal cases. NOT cases are at risk of poor treatment outcomes, such as endur-
ing symptoms after treatment or deterioration, given that their trajectory of
symptoms is markedly different to that of patients with similar characteristics
(Lutz et al., 2006).

In *raw score feedback*, the scores of the patient on the outcome instrument
are plotted in a graph over time, usually together with a cut-off score for normal functioning based on the criteria for clinical significance (Jacobson &
Truax, 1991). Feedback signals are typically provided based on a rule of thumb,
such as a five-point increase in distress compared to the start of treatment (see
Chapter 7 for more details). An example is provided in Figure 1.2, using a

Figure 1.2 Example of raw score feedback

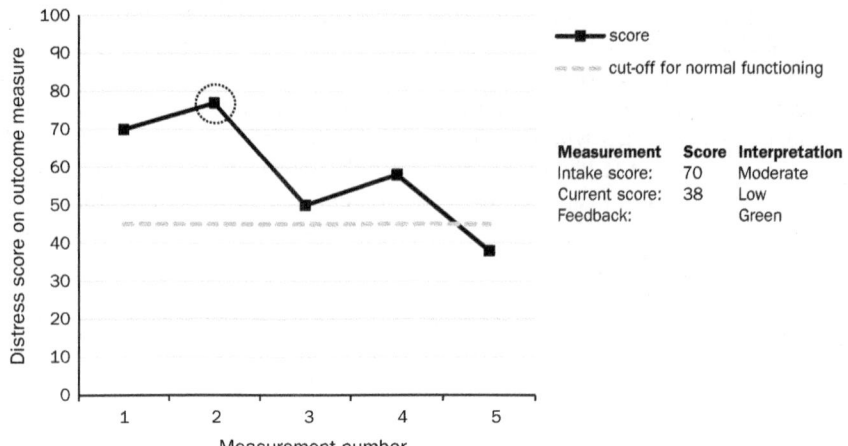

fictional outcome measure with a range between 0 and 100. The score at the start of treatment is 70, which for this instrument is moderate compared to clinical norms for outpatients. At the second session, there has been a seven-point increase in distress, which results in a message to the therapists that the treatment is not-on-track (NOT).

In feedback employing *expected treatment response* (ETR) curves, the score of the patient is benchmarked against a statistical prediction model. The prediction model is typically based on a large database of outcome data from patients previously treated in that service or setting (see more details in Chapter 7). The statistical model generates a failure boundary and positive boundary (see Figure 1.3). The space between these two boundaries represents the measurement fluctuations that are likely to be observed over time. If a measurement crosses the failure boundary, the therapist and/or patient receives a signal that the treatment is not progressing as expected, relative to data from similar patients. In the example, this happens at session 2, where a NOT signal is provided. If the positive boundary is crossed, the therapist receives feedback that the treatment is progressing better than expected.

Feedback that supplements ETR feedback with the use of clinical support tools (CSTs) is referred to as *CST feedback*. Clinical support tools are designed to identify and address problems that might be interfering with treatment progress. The most common way of using CST feedback is that the moment a case is identified as not-on-track (NOT) by the ETR curves, the feedback system prompts patients to complete an additional questionnaire that assesses factors that might be interfering with treatment progress, such as motivational problems, problems in the working alliance between the patient and therapist, problems in coping with stressful life events or, problems related to social support. The instrument assesses if there are problems in these domains and the feedback systems then suggests several interventions – based on the scientific literature – that

Figure 1.3 Example of expected treatment response (ETR) feedback

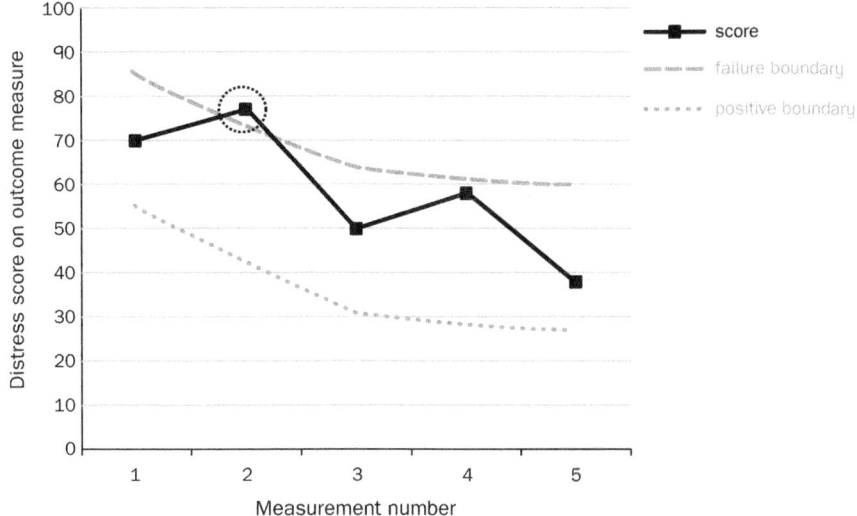

could be employed to address problematic areas. CSTs were initially developed by Michael Lambert's research group (Harmon et al., 2005; 2007; Lambert & Shimokawa, 2011), but have also been used and further developed by other researchers (e.g., Lucock et al., 2015; Lutz et al., 2020).

Why would I need to use ROM?

You may wonder why you would need standardized outcome measures in mental health care. Surely, the therapist should be able to detect if a patient is making progress or not, so why bother patients with completing outcome measures on a regular basis? In response, there are several reasons why it is important to include ROM as part of your practice.

Outcomes in routine care are not that great

Research from the last 50 years has shown that psychological interventions are effective in reducing symptom distress and improving functioning in patients suffering from a wide range of mental health problems (Barkham & Lambert, 2021; De Jong & DeRubeis, 2018). Typically, the effectiveness of psychological interventions is studied in RCTs, and meta-analyses of these studies reveal that approximately between 60 and 70 per cent of patients improve during psychological interventions (Barkham & Lambert, 2021). However, results from routine practice show considerable variability in treatment outcomes and a recovery rate of around 50 per cent has been shown to be a fairly realistic standard (e.g., see Clark, 2018). Hence, there is considerable room for improvement, since one out of two patients may not fully recover from their problems after routinely delivered therapy. Furthermore, research indicates that psychological therapies seem to be slightly less effective for children and young people by comparison to outcomes observed in adults (Ng et al., 2021). While there are some methodological differences between RCTs and results from routine practice that explain a small part of that difference in outcomes, like the strict inclusion criteria that are often applied in RCTs (e.g., Blais et al., 2012), research in the field clearly indicates that many patients do not recover after accessing routinely delivered therapies. Several prominent researchers in the field have suggested that monitoring patients' progress in routine care through the use of standardized measures to inform clinical decision-making is a promising method to improve outcomes in routine care (e.g., Kazdin, 2008; Wampold, 2015).

Therapists are poor at recognizing cases at risk of poor treatment response

Research suggests that therapists are not very good at detecting a lack of progress in their patients or in predicting which patients may not benefit from treatment. Hatfield and colleagues (2010) studied therapists' progress notes to determine whether therapists were able to detect patients who were worsening. From a database with information on over 7000 therapy trajectories, they selected 70 sessions in which patients' symptoms were substantially worsening, as measured by ROM. Yet, in only 21 per cent of the session notes for these sessions, this worsening of symptoms was documented by the therapist.

In a pivotal study, Hannan and colleagues (2005) asked therapists to review their caseload and to identify the patients who they thought might significantly worsen during treatment. The therapists knew that the base rate for these negative outcomes in their practice was 8 per cent. However, in assessing their own case load, therapists thought that their own patients would have a much lower chance of getting negative outcomes. In total, the therapists in the study rated 550 patients and identified only 3 patients (0.5 per cent) who they thought would worsen during treatment. In fact, 40 patients had negative treatment outcomes (7 per cent) and only 1 patient had been correctly identified by the therapists. Hannan and colleagues compared the therapists' assessment with that of a ROM and feedback system that applied ETR models and found that the ETR models could accurately identify 77 per cent of the patients who were not progressing well.

In the study by Hannan et al. (2005), therapists were asked to identify which patients would worsen, which is a fairly rare event. Since it is harder to predict something with a low base rate, in one of our own studies (De Jong et al., in preparation), we asked therapists to identify which of their patients would recover, which would typically be achieved by one-third of the patients in that setting. The results showed that therapists estimated that about two-thirds of patients would recover when no feedback was provided. When ROM and feedback were provided, therapists eventually adjusted their expectations towards a more realistic expectation of patient outcomes.

The results of these studies suggest that therapists have trouble accurately assessing their patients' symptom severity and prognosis. The results also suggest that therapists may overestimate their own treatment outcomes. This is consistent with research by Walfish and colleagues (2012), who asked therapists to rate their own performance compared to their peers. They found that 25 per cent of the therapists ranked themselves among the best 10 per cent in their profession. None rated themselves as below average. This overestimation of oneself is referred to as self-assessment bias (Dunning et al., 2004). It is not unique to psychologists; most people think that they are more intelligent, more attractive and more capable than they objectively are. They also tend to overestimate the odds of positive outcomes and underestimate the odds of negative things happening to them. This may not be such a bad thing, as moderate amounts of positive bias in self-assessment seem to be protective of our mental health. However, more pronounced positive self-bias can lead to unhealthy relationships, engaging in risky behaviours and underperformance (Karpen, 2018). In the context of psychological treatments, it seems important that therapists do not get overly confident about the quality of their treatment, as they might miss that a patient is not progressing well and is at risk of poor treatment outcomes. ROM and feedback have a role in providing therapists with additional information to inform their clinical judgement, and to alert them to cases that are not-on-track.

The scientific evidence: are outcomes enhanced?

Effect on treatment outcomes

By now, a fairly large number of studies have been conducted on the effectiveness of ROM and feedback. Several meta-analytic reviews of clinical trials of feedback-informed treatment have been published since the early 2000s (e.g., Bergman et al., 2018; De Jong et al., 2021; Kendrick et al., 2016; Knaup et al., 2009; Lambert et al., 2003, 2018; Østergård et al., 2020; Pejtersen et al., 2020; Shimokawa et al., 2010; Tam & Ronan, 2017). In the most comprehensive systematic review and meta-analysis to date, we investigated the short and long-term effects of feedback on symptom reduction, the percentage of patients who significantly worsen during treatment, treatment duration, and the percentage of patients who dropout from treatment (De Jong et al., 2021). We synthesized the results from 58 controlled studies, both randomized and non-randomized, analysing a total of 110 effect sizes in studies that included a total of 21,699 patients. The studies were predominantly conducted in adult samples receiving individual outpatient psychological therapies. The majority of studies took place in the United States and Europe. These studies compared the effectiveness of usual psychological care (control groups) versus therapy supplemented by ROM and feedback (experimental groups).

The results showed that there was an overall positive effect of feedback on symptom reduction, relative to usual psychological care without feedback. The effect was both statistically significant and reliable, indicating that feedback demonstrably improves treatment outcomes. While the effect was small in statistical terms (effect size $d = 0.15$), it should be noted that psychological therapies are typically already quite effective in reducing symptoms, with an average effect size of $d = 0.75$–0.85 (Wampold & Imel, 2015), which is interpreted as a large effect. Feedback is an add-on intervention, for which small additional effect sizes should be expected over and above the general effects of therapy. We also found a significant effect of feedback on treatment dropout. The mean dropout rate was 25 per cent in control groups and 21 per cent in feedback groups, which indicates that feedback utilization helps to reduce dropout. The feedback had no significant effect on the percentage of deteriorated cases or on the duration of treatment.

Subgroup analyses were conducted for NOT cases. We would expect feedback to have the largest effects in NOT cases, since feedback-using therapists are more likely to make changes in the treatment to prevent poor outcomes. This difference in effectiveness was indeed found in earlier meta-analyses (Kendrick et al., 2016; Lambert et al., 2018; Shimokawa et al., 2010), but not in ours. We found a similar effect of feedback in NOT subgroup ($d = 0.17$) as in the full sample. Hence, we conclude from this that feedback is not only helpful in situations where therapy is not going well, but it can also enhance treatment progress in cases that are on track to a positive outcome.

Factors that influence the effectiveness of ROM and feedback

There are substantial differences between studies and feedback systems, so in the above-mentioned meta-analysis we wanted to take a closer look at whether these variables also influenced the effectiveness of the feedback. A few factors were found to influence one or more types of treatment outcomes (symptom reduction, dropout, deterioration, and treatment duration), namely the type of feedback used, the feedback instrument, the frequency of the measurements, and treatment intensity. In addition, it was found that the effects of feedback were larger in the United States than in other countries. This might be caused by a number of factors, such as cultural differences, differences in professional training, and health care systems, as well as access to care.

The most influential predictors were the type of feedback and the feedback instrument(s). These factors are somewhat entangled, because feedback systems typically offer feedback on one specific outcome measure. The two most studied feedback systems are PCOMS and the OQ System, together accounting for more than two-thirds of the studies. PCOMS consists of a measure of functioning, the Outcome Rating Scale (ORS; Miller et al., 2003), and an assessment of the therapeutic alliance, the Session Rating Scale (SRS; Duncan et al., 2003). The OQ System consists of a combination of the Outcome Questionnaire (OQ; Lambert et al., 2004) and clinical support tools. While a variety of other feedback systems are available (see Table 2.4, Chapter 2), these have often not been studied in a controlled way in more than a few studies. In the meta-analysis, it was found that PCOMS was the most effective feedback system for patients who were progressing well compared to the OQ and other feedback systems, whereas the OQ System with CST feedback was most effective in not-on-track cases (De Jong et al., 2021).

A factor that could not be assessed directly in the meta-analysis, but is known to influence the effectiveness of feedback, is the degree of implementation (e.g., see Bickman et al., 2016; De Jong et al., 2012; Simon et al., 2012). Service-wide implementation of ROM and feedback can be challenging for a variety of reasons, a topic we discuss in more detail in Chapter 3.

Differential effects due to the context of care

A factor that is worth noting, is that research has found some differential effects of feedback with respect to the context of treatment. Individual studies have shown that feedback can have an effect on symptom reduction, treatment duration (or the efficiency of treatment), and dropout, but typically these effects are not all found at the same time. In some services, feedback will improve symptom reduction and reduce the number of deteriorated cases, whereas in other services, the efficiency of treatment is enhanced. The latter typically occurs when services work in a more standardized way or have relatively good outcomes already before the implementation of ROM and feedback.

Cost-effectiveness

Although the research on the cost-effectiveness of ROM and feedback has only just started, it is worth mentioning here, as this might be an important factor for policy makers and health care services. In a recent study on the effectiveness of feedback, the cost-effectiveness of ROM and feedback was assessed for the first time. The study took place within several IAPT services in England and feedback improved the percentage of reliably improved patients by 8 percentage points at only a slight incremental cost of £15.17 per treatment. This suggests that better outcomes can be achieved at a slightly higher cost, which suggests that ROM and feedback is cost-effective (Delgadillo et al., 2021).

Conclusions

As a field, we have come a long way since the early 1900s in outcome measurement. Which is clearly a good thing, considering that as human beings, we are not that good at accurately assessing risks. Thus, without help, therapists may not be able to detect which patients are at risk for poor treatment outcomes. ROM and feedback methods have been developed to help therapists to detect these cases early in treatment and there is now robust evidence that this improves psychological treatment outcomes and reduces dropout. While the current chapter is more theoretical, the remainder of this book is more practical, aimed at helping therapists to select outcome measures, to interpret these measures, to discuss these measures with patients, and to integrate ROM and feedback in routine practice and clinical supervision.

Key points in this chapter

- Outcome measures can be used in different ways and to fulfill different goals that matter to patients, therapists, services, researchers, funders, and policy makers.
- Psychological treatment outcomes in routine clinical practice are highly variable and sometimes less optimistic than those observed in clinical trials.
- It is difficult for therapists to assess whether or not patients are benefitting from treatment. ROM and feedback help with this difficult task.
- ROM and feedback help to improve clinical outcomes and to reduce treatment dropout in a cost-effective way.

Endnote

1 As of January 2023, the UK Improving Access to Psychological Therapies (IAPT) programme that is referred to in the text has been renamed as 'NHS Talking Therapies for Anxiety and Depression'. For familiarity, we have retained the term IAPT in the text.

2 Principles for selecting ROM and feedback tools for your practice

In this chapter

In this chapter, we provide an overview of the principles and procedures for selecting and implementing outcome measures and feedback systems. The chapter describes five key domains of decision-making, covering considerations about response burden, relevance and accessibility, psychometric properties, sensitivity to change, and cost. It contains a brief primer on basic concepts in the field of psychometrics, which may be informative to readers unfamiliar with this area of psychology. For readers who are already versed in psychometrics, we offer a discussion on the trade-offs between the above five domains, which should be considered when deciding how to integrate measurement into clinical practice.

Measuring, monitoring, or obtaining feedback?

A first decision point in working with ROM and feedback is whether you want to measure outcomes, monitor outcomes or use feedback (see Chapter 1). As some of you may already use outcome measurement of some kind, we want to outline briefly why we think that moving to a ROM and feedback system might be more beneficial for patients, therapists, and services.

A key principle of good practice is that any information collected needs to be of value to the patient, therapist, and organization. While outcome measurement is of value to organizations (e.g., for evaluation and benchmarking purposes), it typically does not add much value for the therapist and patient, as in many situations they do not get to see the results. Thus, measurement is often used as a source of administrative information rather than as a data source to inform treatment decisions. Even if results are available to therapists and patients, a low frequency of measurements (e.g., before and after therapy) may make it hard to integrate such information into the treatment plan, given that each measurement has some degree of measurement error and is a momentary assessment of how the patient is functioning and feeling at that particular time. Another drawback of an infrequent outcome measurement system is that there is often a lot of missing data for multiple patients on the post-treatment measurement. Many patients decide, for a variety of reasons, not to continue with therapy and it is then very difficult to obtain sufficient data in this situation such that it can reliably represent all patients. In addition, therapists forget to administer the measurement and patients are sometimes no longer motivated to complete a measurement after treatment. The result is that a service may only have complete data (pre and post therapy) for a small portion of their patients, making the data much less useful for quality assurance purposes and also making it harder to interpret the summarized outcomes of a service. This is because we do not know whether data is missing at random after treatment (less problematic) or whether it is systematic; for instance, if missing data is a result only of people who left the treatment prematurely because they were not progressing (more problematic). From a research perspective, only having two measurement points limits our ability to understand how patients change over time during treatment. With pre-post treatment measurements, only a linear relationship – a straight line – can be modelled, which makes it harder to understand the process of change, and we know from research that treatment progress is often not linear, but rather shows large improvements in the beginning of treatment and smaller improvements after the initial change (see Figure 2.1).

So, there are good reasons to move from measurement to monitoring. The question is then: can any outcome measure also be used for monitoring and feedback purposes? The answer to that is probably both yes and no. In principle, any measure can be used routinely, but in practice, more frequent administration of an outcome measure creates some restrictions due to issues relating to the length, costs, administrative burden and ease of use, and interpretation of the instrument. Especially when using an outcome measure for feedback, it is crucial that results are easy to understand for both the patient and the therapist. This can be an issue as, historically, many of the outcome measures available to therapists and services were designed as outcome measures rather than

Figure 2.1 Modelling data from outcome measurement versus outcome monitoring

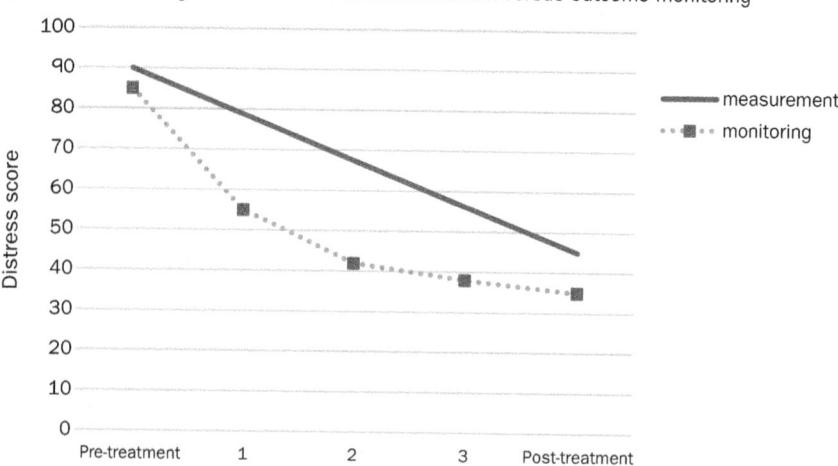

monitoring or feedback measures. In the next section, we consider a number of issues relating to the choice of a monitoring and feedback measure and the impact they have on the decision-making process.

Key considerations in choosing a monitoring and feedback measure

In choosing a measure for monitoring and feedback, one important point needs to be taken into consideration: the majority of available outcome measures have not been designed with an integrative view of assessment followed by repeated frequent use. Hence, to select measures for monitoring and feedback, therapists are currently adopting some measures designed for a different purpose. This is not to invalidate any of the available measures; but it is important to recognize this limitation. There have been a few measures that have been developed from a monitoring and feedback perspective, but some of these still lean heavily on traditional outcome measurement methodology in how they are scored and interpreted. With that point in mind, we can now turn to outline the five main considerations when selecting a measure. A summary of these key considerations is provided in Table 2.1.

Length and burden

The length of the measure is a major factor in repeated administrations, and particularly when the measure is administered at every session. There are no widely agreed rules or criteria about the set number of items that a

Table 2.1 Five key considerations in choosing and adopting a feedback measure

Criterion	Key question(s)
Length and burden	Are the number of items and time taken to complete the measure likely to be burdensome?
Relevance and accessibility	Is the measure appropriate for the patient group and setting? Are validated translations available in other languages?
Psychometric properties	Does it have established psychometric properties such as validity, reliability, reliable change/clinical significance/norms?
Sensitivity to change	Is the measure sensitive enough to capture changes experienced during therapy?
Costs, copyright, and Creative Commons	Is a licence required to use the measure? Is it affordable?

questionnaire should ideally have. As an observation, there has been a recent momentum towards measures comprising in the region of 10 items when used at every session, but this should not be construed as a rule or reason to exclude consideration of measures containing a higher number of items.

While it might be attractive to get a very brief instrument in order to reduce the burden on the patient, an instrument that is too short typically has lower reliability and lower sensitivity to change (see next sections). In effect, the oft-used principle of the measure being 'fit for purpose' is a reasonable axiom to use. Hence, if on the basis of initial piloting (see later) it is found that some people are not completing the measure due to fatigue, then this would be a reason to re-evaluate using that specific measure. Similarly, if people were missing out selected items, again, this would be a reason to investigate what was leading to this outcome. The guiding principle should be that the task, when repeated, does not become aversive or a barrier to patients returning for therapy – that would defeat the objective.

What might be more important than the number of items of a measure is the time needed to complete it. This is a function of both the number of items and the complexity of the items (i.e., because of the wording or level of detail required). When patients complete the measure regularly, they will typically get faster in completing it over time, especially if they complete it every session. Do take into account that therapists and researchers tend to underestimate how long it takes patients to complete measures and how much of a burden they are. The comment by a patient below is illustrative of this fact.

> "I had not imagined that completing a questionnaire could be so painful to me, but it confronted me with how poorly I was feeling and functioning and I found it quite hard to complete in the beginning of treatment."
> — Anonymous patient, the Netherlands

This comment may also be understandable in light of the ambivalence that many patients are feeling when entering treatment. While they might be happy to get help, it also means that they are functioning so poorly that they cannot resolve it on their own.

Relevance, accessibility, and diversity considerations

Relevance and accessibility refer, in many ways, to the face validity of the measures from the viewpoint of both the service and the patient. When administering the same measure at a high frequency it is good to keep in mind that the purpose is not to provide a full assessment, but rather an assessment that provides the most important information for monitoring progress that can be administered in a short time period.

> "The questionnaires that were used were quite short so I did not feel that they were capturing an enormous amount. It felt like there were things missing from

them, sometimes my answers did not really reflect how I had been feeling, but I appreciate having brief measures is very useful for keeping track of progress".
— Anonymous patient, UK.

Accessibility refers to the extent to which a questionnaire makes sense to a respondent, is easily understandable and is thus less likely to lead to invalid responses. There are several diversity issues to consider in selecting an outcome measure. When selecting measures, it is important to consider if the wording (e.g., use of jargon or unusual words) and format (e.g., use of Likert scales or other scoring schemes) are likely to be understandable to the target clinical population. For instance, children and young people may require questionnaires that have been specifically designed to be appropriate to their reading age and developmental stage. The availability of translated measures into different languages is also an important consideration to enable services to be inclusive and accessible to people from different sociocultural backgrounds. It has been well documented that cultural differences can influence the way in which people complete a questionnaire. Not all outcome measures are culturally sensitive, so it is important to consider your target patient population and to think about whether the items might be interpreted differently by people from another cultural background. Similarly, some items about interpersonal and relational functioning, which is a common area to measure in ROM, are formulated from the perspective of heterosexual relationships, which may not be inclusive for people with different gender and sexual orientations. Such aspects of diversity and inclusion should be carefully considered by therapists and services when deciding on which measures to use.

Short forms versus original measures

Some measures used for monitoring and feedback have been developed as a short form of an originally longer version of a well-established outcome measure. Choosing a measure that has an empirical relationship with a more comprehensive assessment has the advantage that the longer instrument could be used at intake to get a broad assessment of symptoms and functioning, and the short form could be used for monitoring, and one would still, for instance, have information on the same subdomains. Examples of such a combination of measures include the following: the Brief Symptom Inventory (BSI; Derogatis, 1977), which is the short form of the Symptom Checklist-Revised-90 (SCL-R-90; Derogatis, 1975), and the ASEBA Brief Problem Monitor (Achenbach et al., 2011), which is the short form of the Child Behavior Checklist (CBCL; Achenbach, 1991). A potential downside of using short forms is that they are often, but not always, licensed and entail a cost to purchase.

Specific, generic, and multi-domain measures

One key dimension in the choice of a measure is the extent to which an instrument focuses on a specific condition or captures a greater bandwidth of dimensions in a person's life. Hence, measures can be grouped into those that focus on a defined condition (specific) versus those that are generic. The choice involves a number of factors that balance providing a clear and reliable signal of change but also, in effect, narrowing the focus of outcome monitoring. For example, the choice of a single measure of depression might enable an adequate process of outcome monitoring in that specific domain, but it also narrows the monitoring process to that single domain. Put another way, the content of the measure presents a strong message of what the treatment is focusing on. If the repeated measure focuses on depression, is this the only or most relevant domain for that patient? Might a patient think that the service is only interested in the level of their depression? A potential downside of using a single specific measure is that symptoms may shift over time. For example, a patient might present with depressive symptoms at the start of treatment, but after a few sessions, more and more anxious symptoms start to emerge. The therapist would then need to switch or include additional measures, otherwise they would not have much information on the anxious symptoms. Nevertheless, there are situations where a specific measure and monitoring process would be entirely appropriate and would minimize response burden; such as in specialist services for a specific condition (e.g., a specialist clinic for obsessive-compulsive disorder, birth-related trauma, or prolonged grief disorder, etc.).

By contrast, generic measures aim to capture broader dimensions of people's lives such as their wellbeing, level of functioning, relationships, social activities, etc. Measures that are not tied to a single presenting condition and yet yield an index that could be valuable for ongoing monitoring might focus on *functioning*. One of the simplest indices of functioning is the Global Assessment of Functioning (GAF), in which a person locates themselves at a point on a 1–100 scale. Another measure is the five-item Work and Social Adjustment Scale (WSAS; Mundt et al., 2002), which has been used as part of the Minimum Data Set within the Improving Access to Psychological Therapies (IAPT) programme. Regardless of whether a person is experiencing depression, anxiety, obsessive thoughts, etc., how they are functioning may provide a valuable index capturing the extent to which they are coping with life in general. Another construct that can enable monitoring of wider aspects of a person's functioning is that of *quality of life* (QoL). QoL measures have a long tradition in the areas of physical health, but there is an increasing literature based on aspects of quality of life within the area of the psychological therapies. One example is a 10-item measure termed Recovering Quality of Life (ReQoL; Keetharuth et al., 2018).

Examples of multi-domain assessment measures that capture a broader range of aspects include the following: Outcome Questionnaire (OQ-45.2; Lambert et al., 2004); Partners for Change Outcome Management System (PCOMS; Miller et al., 2005); Counseling Center Assessment of Psychological Symptoms (CCAPS; Locke et al., 2011); Clinical Outcomes in Routine Evaluation measures – CORE-OM (Evans et al., 2002), CORE-10 (Barkham et al., 2013); Treatment Outcome Package (TOP; Kraus, & Castonguay, 2010); CelestHealth – Behavioral Health Measure-20 (BHM-20; Kopta et al., 2015). However, by definition, it is likely that a measure sampling a broader scope of presenting problems will lead to more items. An overview of commonly used generic instruments that are used for monitoring and feedback is presented in Table 2.4. at the end of this chapter. The choice of selecting a single specific measure, a generic measure, a multi-domain measure, or some combination of measures should depend on the service's target population. For example, a battery of measures covering various specific symptom-domains could be used as a repository to select a specific measure depending on each patient's presenting problem(s). Such a targeted measure could then be supplemented by a more generic measure of functioning, or a multi-domain measure that also captures important aspects of interpersonal functioning and risk. In general, the more information a therapist has, the better able they will be to track progress and to adjust the treatment plan in a personalised way. However, this ideal scenario (multiple measures) has to be balanced against response burden.

> *"What has struck me as the most important thing to be mindful of in the development of a feedback system is that, from the patient's perspective, by asking them certain questions, we are also telling them something about what we find relevant for the therapeutic context. There is meta-communication through the measures and systems that you use about what your clinical interest is. So, we need to be mindful that the system is welcoming a breath of experiences. Patients are very attentive to its relevance and see the feedback system as a proxy for the health care provider and reflect on whether this provider would fit their needs and can address their core concerns. A natural implication of this, in my opinion, is that we need to allow quite a wide area of experiences to be measured within the feedback system."*
>
> Christian Moltu – emotion-focused therapist and
> feedback researcher, Norway

Risk and safety

One key component to consider in selecting a measure relates to monitoring risk and ensuring patient safety. It is important to decide if the measure to be selected enables risk monitoring or, if not, how this crucial aspect is going to be included in any feedback system. There is an argument that for many, if not all patients, the initial assessment should gather information about risks to self or others. Of course, this can be achieved through dialogue, but a service should consider whether this domain is one that they wish to be included in an outcome monitoring system. With shorter measures, it is likely that there may be a single item capturing some aspects of risk; for example, thoughts or plans related to self-harm or suicide (e.g., PHQ-9; CORE-10).

Diversity issues

There are several diversity issues to consider in selecting an outcome measure. It has been well reported that cultural differences can influence response patterns on questionnaires (e.g., Kemmelmeier, 2016). Not all outcome measures are culturally sensitive, so it is important to consider your own patient population and think about whether the items might be interpreted differently by people from varying cultural backgrounds. Similarly, items about interpersonal functioning, which is a common area to measure in ROM, are formulated from a heteronormative perspective. For example, questions asking about attractions to people of the opposite sex might not be relevant to ask participants who identify as bisexual or gay.

Basic psychometrics and features

Validity and reliability

The psychometric properties of any measure are, in effect, its credentials in terms of showing whether it has scientific credibility. The standard considerations are those of validity and reliability. All instrument developers will report on these constructs: does it measure what it purports to measure (validity)? Does it consistently measure the same construct each time (reliability)? The basic components of validity and reliability are summarized in Tables 2.2 and 2.3 respectively. While this may sound relatively straightforward, there is one key point to keep in mind, namely, that reported psychometrics will be a function of the population sampled and there can be no guarantee that the stated properties generalize from one population to another. However, it is likely that more widely adopted measures will report data that should provide evidence showing whether the properties of a measure are sufficiently stable across settings and populations.

Table 2.2 Components of measurement validity

Validity type	Explanation
Construct validity	Construct validity can be viewed as the central component of validity – it addresses the issue of whether the instrument measures what it purports to measure. Hence, if the target measure is of depression, is it measuring depression only or is it capturing other presentations (e.g., anxiety)? Some aspects are more nuanced; for example, if the measure asks about self-worth, is this a feature of depression or is the measure as a whole more about self-worth? Construct validity is the overarching component regarding validity.
Face validity	Face validity is the simplest form of evaluating how the construct being measured is understood by the intended respondents. If someone is completing a measure of depression, will *they* view it as a questionnaire about depression? It is an evaluation based on the measure's face value: 'On the face of it, it seems to measure depression'. This is clearly a judgement and likely to be viewed as the weakest form of evidence for validity. However, if the depression measure was presented to 10 experts in the field of depression and they all said that, on the face of it, the measure appeared to be measuring the construct of depression, then this evidence would give credibility to the face validity of the measure.

Table 2.2 *(Continued)*

Validity type	Explanation
Criterion validity	Criterion validity evaluates the degree to which a measure corresponds to an established 'gold standard' measure of the same construct. So, again, using depression as an example, a measure of depression might be evaluated against a diagnostic assessment of depression or against a well-established depression measure in the literature. Of course, it might be expected that better criterion validity will arise where there is no method variance (i.e., method invariance); so, testing a self-report measure against another self-report measure may be better than comparing a self-report with a clinical assessment procedure where it would not be expected to obtain as high criterion validity due to the different methods (i.e., method variance).
Content validity	Content validity speaks to the issue of whether the measure captures the full range of the phenomenon or construct under investigation. Again, considering depression, does the measure capture all the differing manifestations of depression (e.g., cognitive, emotional, behavioural, etc.)? Similarly, if the measure is capturing psychological distress, does it cover all the major aspects of psychological distress? In this context, it can be seen that the broader the construct being measured is (e.g., psychological distress), the more likely it is that this will require a greater number of items, resulting in a longer measure. However, choosing to select a shorter measure may result in a highly specific rather than broad measure.
Predictive validity	Predictive validity addresses the ability of a measure to predict a state or condition at some point in the future. This form of validity is likely to be more relevant to screening activities in order to identify the future health status of a person. In our example of depression, a measure will capture the current status and so the predictive element of such a measure would be whether specific scores or profile of scores might, for example, correlate with future levels of depression severity or specific aspects of depression (e.g., greater vulnerability to self-harm).
Discriminant validity	Discriminant validity has two components: convergent validity and divergent validity. Put simply, convergent validity relates to associations with other measures that would be expected to be measuring the same construct (e.g., other measures of depression) while divergent validity would be assessed by evaluating the association with a different construct (e.g., anxiety). Hence, the magnitude of associations (i.e., correlations) between a measure of depression should be stronger with other depression measures and weaker with measures of anxiety (but there will be an association due to the expected comorbidity between depression and anxiety).

Table 2.3 Components of measurement reliability

Reliability type	Explanation
Internal reliability	Internal reliability – also referred to as internal consistency – focuses on the reliability of the measure in itself (i.e., at the same time point); examples are: split-half reliability and alpha coefficient.
Split-half reliability	Split-half reliability seeks to establish the comparative reliabilities when a measure is split into two halves; the procedure for splitting could be based on any principle (e.g., alternate items; first half vs latter half; or at random). This method assumes that the two halves of the test should yield similar results (e.g., scores and error variances), if indeed the items are all measuring a common underlying construct.
Alpha reliability	Alpha reliability determines how closely interrelated a set of items are as a group, and it is commonly measured using Cronbach's alpha coefficient. The higher this coefficient (ranging from 0 to 1, expressed in decimals), the higher the internal consistency of items (i.e., they are strongly interrelated and thus measure a common underlying construct).
External reliability	External reliability focuses on consistency across time; an example is test-retest reliability.
Test-retest reliability	Test-retest reliability establishes the stability of the measure over time. The test-retest reliability can be time specific (e.g., 1-week reliability, 2 weeks, 1 month, etc.). The stronger the index of correlation between repeated measures, the greater the evidence of test-retest reliability. Such repeated measures are often taken at short intervals (e.g., 1 week) and in the absence of treatment in order to establish how reliable a questionnaire is to measure the level of a condition that is presumably stable during the observation period.

Reliable change and clinical significance

Reliable change and *clinical significance* are concepts that have been developed in order to make it easier to interpret the change score of an individual patient in a meaningful way (Jacobson & Truax, 1991). Reliable change refers to the amount of change that is beyond the measurement error of the instrument, and therefore might reliably reflect change that is statistically reliable and not simply due to chance or error. Clinical significance refers to the clinical status of a patient relative to a cut-off score that differentiates between clinical and sub-clinical levels of symptoms or distress. These two components of reliable change and clinical significance have been widely adopted in the field of psychotherapy research and practice (Evans et al., 1998) and will be discussed in more detail in Chapter 6. For the selection of outcome measures, it is important to determine whether these indices are available for the outcome measure of choice, and to keep in mind that these indices are influenced by the clinical populations and samples that were collected for the original psychometric evaluation of the measure. Samples should be both sufficiently large and relevant to the population you are aiming to measure.

Test norms

Test norms are data that make it possible to compare the score of a patient to a group of individuals, typically a 'clinical' group and a 'non-clinical' group, in order to determine the relative functioning of the patient. By itself, the raw score of a patient often has little meaning, unless the score is located at the extremes (i.e., very low or very high). This procedure is rooted in the notion of *social comparisons* in which the outcomes of an individual or of a group of individuals are compared against known outcomes from other studies that enable statements to be made about the extent and impact of the any given outcome (e.g., Nietzel et al., 1987). Typically, the score of the patient is compared to a percentile score, which refers to the comparison group's percentage of individuals falling below that score. So, if a patient's score at intake is at the 75th percentile compared to an outpatient population, it means that 75 per cent of outpatients typically score below this score, therefore indicating that the patient is suffering to a considerable degree. What is important to review in a test manual when selecting an outcome measure is that the normative groups are large enough (typically at least 300 subjects per group) and that the sample comprises sufficient patients from the population you are targeting in your service. For example, if you are aiming to measure outcomes in an inpatient setting, the measure should have collected a sample in that specific setting. In addition, it is good to realize that norms are sometimes collected in a predominantly white heterosexual sample, which may make them less useful for diverse populations, such as minorities.

Timeframe

One property on which measures can be distinguished concerns whether they are capturing an individual's current state or change in their state. The vast majority of measures focus on state – how a person has been over some specified period of time. This is akin to taking a photo (or an elapsed time photo) that captures a person's state. The other approach is where a measure asks the patient to state how much things have changed over some specified time period. While the focus on change would appear to be exactly what a practitioner is wanting to find out, the format introduces each patient as a separate and different measuring mechanism. It is akin to providing an answer to a maths question without showing the original data or the calculations. Accordingly, we would advise against measures that use this latter format.

In terms of the specified period of time (e.g., *How you have been over the past [week] [two weeks] [month]?*), it is likely that whatever timeframe is used in a measure, patients' responses will be weighted according to how they feel now. Because of this, and because of difficulties in recalling feelings and experiences going back in time, a one-week time frame probably has advantages over longer time periods. In addition, many (but by no means all) patients have weekly sessions, and having a one-week timeline for the sessional measure makes a good fit. Where sessions are weekly and the measure is capturing information from a longer time period, it is likely that some patients may misinterpret the timeline and complete it as covering the time since they last completed the measure. This point also has a bearing on the next issue.

A potential interpretation problem arises when more than a single session is captured within the timeframe of a measure. There are two scenarios where this can happen. The first is where a practitioner sees a patient more than once a week, which is more common these days as it can increase the effectiveness of the treatment (e.g., Reese et al., 2011). The second is where sessions are weekly but the timeframe of the measure is longer (e.g., monthly). In both these situations, there will be an overlap in the sampling time of the measures such that successive measures will be sampling some of the same time period.

Sensitivity to change

Beyond the basic issues of validity and reliability, the key criterion for any measure is *sensitivity to change* and this probably is even more important when adopting ROM and feedback. Establishing reliable weekly estimates of change puts a high demand on a measure as it is being expected to identify, reliably, more granular change over the course of time rather than a direct comparison between two time points multiple weeks or more apart (as in traditional pre–post treatment comparisons). A corollary of this point is the need to ensure that repeated measures are not susceptible to 'floor and ceiling effects'. A floor effect refers to a situation where a measure is not sensitive enough to capture different gradients of low-level severity, whereas a ceiling effect refers to an inability to capture different gradients of high-level severity. For instance, if a measure shows a maximum score at one session and the same maximum score at the next session, this measure appears to be indicating no change. However, it may be that change has occurred but the instrument is not sufficiently sensitive to show it due to ceiling effects, thereby undermining the utility of the measure.

The sensitivity to change requirement is for a measure to show both real and reliable change repeatedly. By *real* change, we mean that the data needs to match clinical observations. This is by no means a perfect science; some patients mask their feelings, which leads to discrepancies between reported data and a patient's presentation. In a comparison of group-level data, the tendency of some patients to under-report and others to over-report specific items cancel each other out. However, if the data is used at an individual level, then such influences on the reporting of a clinical state and change become important – that is, they need to be reliable if they are to be used to inform treatment.

An instrument's sensitivity to change is determined by the content of the instrument, but also by the scoring range, with larger scoring ranges typically showing larger sensitivity to change. As a result, measures with more items and larger answering scales (i.e., seven-point scale) tend to have a higher sensitivity to change.

Costs, copyright, and licences

A final consideration, although for some it may be the first, concerns the cost of the selected measure and issues of copyright. While not promoting any specific outcome measure, we are clear that, in the context of many outcome measures being free, it is a challenge to justify the spend on the actual measures themselves (although such costs may be covered by insurance arrangements). However, some measurement systems provide support in the interpretation of measures and such a facility justifies the costs. One reasoned position is that access to the actual measures themselves should be free in order for therapists working alone or in less developed systems to be able to access the measures for a no or lo-tech approach to ROM and clinical feedback.

I chose the questionnaire I am using now because it is free of charge and it comes from a trusted source – it was developed by our local university. It is reliable and valid, but still needs to be normed. Furthermore, a questionnaire has to be easy to use, so that I can read the graphs easily. I prefer a short questionnaire with a global score. As a private practitioner, I am not specialised in only one type of disorder, but I see a wide range of patients. I work in specialised mental health care, so patients often have several DSM classifications; a specific questionnaire is complicated then. I'm not just interested in symptoms reduction, I also want my patients to feel better and have fewer disabilities. If all of that is included in a questionnaire, I find that attractive.

– Erik van der Put, private practitioner and CBT therapist, the Netherlands

Monitoring other domains than outcome

It will be evident that ROM is focused on outcomes and these can extend beyond symptoms (e.g., functioning, quality of life). But they can also include contextual and process elements, and several feedback systems also include measures of context and processes in their monitoring system. For example, patients approach therapy with a range of differing expectations; some patients are expecting it to change their lives while others attend reluctantly and have virtually no expectation of therapy helping at all (Constantino et al., 2011). Hence, monitoring the patient's expectations seems empirically and clinically appropriate. Similarly, there is a literature on stages of change that talks about states of patient readiness and motivation to change (Prochaska & DiClemente, 1983). These aspects of motivation can also be monitored and targeted as a focus for therapeutic work. Other processes such as the working alliance are well-documented predictors of treatment outcomes (Flückiger et al., 2019). Being able to monitor and focus on these elements may provide a route to securing better overall outcomes, and are also likely to enable a patient to remain in therapy as opposed to dropping out. The message here, perhaps, is that there is a need to monitor, albeit in a way that minimizes response burden, key aspects of the therapeutic process in addition to outcome indicators, rather than only being driven by a desire to achieve a good score on a specific outcome measure.

The practicalities of using ROM

Measurement frequency

Importantly, ROM does not necessarily mean taking a measure at every session. If the rationale is to maximize the generation of data, then measuring outcomes at every session would be the strategy to adopt. Such a strategy would enable the identification of session-by-session changes that potentially provide the most information to practitioners and service managers. It is also the easiest to implement as there is no question whether this particular session has a ROM or not; all sessions have a ROM. And it is certainly true that such a strategy has yielded very large datasets for researchers in the field of the psychological therapies and, to the extent that the outputs from these datasets help improve services, then this strategy has much to recommend it. A clear example of this approach is the work arising from the English IAPT programme (e.g., see systematic review by Wakefield et al., 2021).

However, there are points to consider before adopting this strategy relating to the use of the data and the patient population. Regarding use of the data, it is a fair premise that data of any kind should not be collected gratuitously – that is, without good reason. In short, if data is collected at every session, it needs to be used, initially and primarily by the practitioner. And the type of use can vary: it can be used as a summary (i.e., total score); identification of individual items to highlight change (or no change), each of which can be addressed in the form of clinical feedback to the patient; and it can be used as the basis for a dialogic approach to the content and focus on the subsequent therapy session.

The other consideration is the patient population. While gathering data at every session when treatment durations are upwards of 20 sessions or slightly more, then session-by-session data collection is well established. But if the intervention is long-term therapy, or if the person is an in-patient, then in such situations, is taking a measure at every session the best strategy? Where the planned treatment or context is one of longer-term therapy, the yield from session-by-session measurement needs to be considered. One option is to administer ROM once a month (e.g., the first meeting in any month). However, a blended approach in which weekly measures (or at every session if not weekly) are adopted in the early phase of therapy and then moved to monthly is another option. The reasoning for such a front-loaded implementation is that many of the key components of therapy need to be established early on; for example, ensuring engagement in therapy, developing an effective working alliance, establishing a routine, etc. In addition, often a disproportionate amount of change occurs early in therapy and having access to sessional data could make a significant contribution to understanding this initial process of engagement in therapy.

The principle of using ROM in service of therapy is that there is a *fit* between the activity and the yield such that ROM becomes integrated with the therapy. As suggested above, there are some models of delivery where taking ROM at every session is a good fit, but there may be others where it is not.

Measuring before, after, or during the session?

There are a number of options as to when patients can complete the designated outcome measure: they can complete it before they arrive at the session, on arrival but before the start of the session, during the session, at the end of the session, or take it away and complete it at home. Key factors in influencing when to have the form completed are (a) standardization, and (b) maximizing the utility of the information. Standardization requires the same procedure to be used on all occasions. Measuring before or after the session at home results in the largest variance in when the measures are being administered, which is not ideal, but in some settings it might be the best option (e.g., in services that do not have a waiting area, or in group therapy, when the measurement reports for the whole group need to be available at the start of the session). Completing the measure upon arrival, immediately prior to the session, typically in the waiting area, is the most commonly adopted time frame, as it makes the information provided by the measure immediately available to inform the start of the session. Some feedback systems require completing the measures in the session, together with the therapists. This has the advantage that it is immediately used as a communication tool and completion rates are typically very high in those cases. The downside is that this is only feasible for very short measures, as it would otherwise take too much time from the session. Another disadvantage of in-session completion is that it may promote socially desirable answers.

Mode of administration

The mode of administration of ROM is a key practical focus that reflects issues of resources. In effect, this is about a no-, lo-, or hi-tech approach to data collection and use.

- The *no-tech* mode uses what has always been termed a 'paper and pencil' approach. Such an approach can often be the simplest for therapists working alone and, importantly, will be familiar to all patients. However, while the interface with patients is with paper and pencil, the therapist will need to transfer the data into some simple system, such as a spreadsheet which allows simple analyses, charts, and graphs to be generated.
- The *lo-tech* mode might involve the use of tablets or some standard digital device for data collection, which again can be transferred to a spreadsheet. But the key point here is that the interface with the patient uses technology that most, if not all, patients are now aware of and are likely to be able to use. But, of course, this needs to be checked with each person as it is important that the presentation of such digital devices does not create a barrier to participation in ROM.
- The *hi-tech* mode represents a shift to fully computerized, and most often commercial, systems in which the interface will be with a digital device or computer that then generates outputs for the therapist that can be shared with patients.

In choosing between these modes of administration, the costs of the system and ease of use are important considerations. Hi-tech monitoring can be costly, but since processes are more automated, may save costs in manual labour, particularly for larger services. Another advantage of hi-tech systems is that they can offer the more advanced types of feedback systems more easily, such as expected treatment response curves and clinical support tools. For smaller practices and services, hi-tech systems may be too expensive (this depends on the licensing system of the software organization), and lo-tech or no-tech solutions might be a better option. Importantly, whatever level of technology and mode of administration is used, the priority should also focus on the process of engagement with the patient and subsequently on making best use of the collected data to inform and improve clinical decision-making. Figure 2.2 provides a decision tree that can aid decision-making on mode of administration and measurement frequency.

Figure 2.2 Decision tree on selecting a mode of administration and measurement frequency

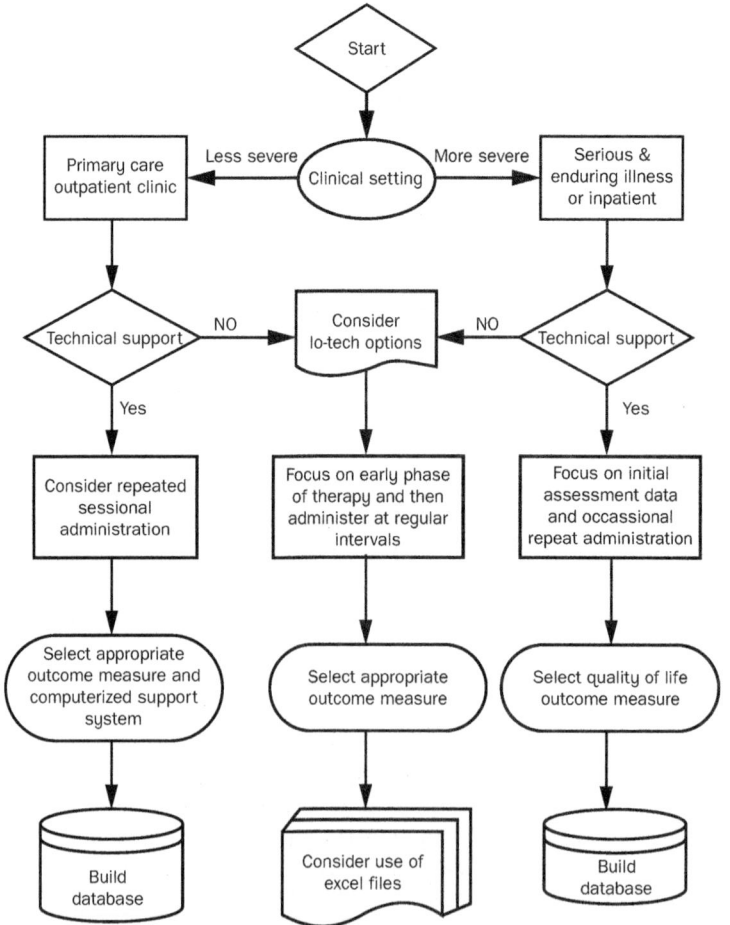

Table 2.4 Ten current ROM/clinical feedback measures/systems

System/Measure(s)	Key source/references		Website(s)
Behavioral Health Measure-20 (BHM-20)	Kopta et al. (2015)	Adults	https://www.celesthealth.com/instruments.asp
Counseling Center Assessment of Psychological Symptoms (CCAPS)	Locke et al. (2011)	Adults	https://ccmh.psu.edu/ccaps-34-62
Common Factors Feedback (CFF)	McClintock et al. (2017)	Adults	
Contextualized Feedback Systems (CFS)	Bickman et al. (2016)	Youth	
CORE System	Barkham et al. (2015)	Adults	https://www.coresystemtrust.org.uk/ https://www.coreims.co.uk/
OQ-45.2 and Y-OQ 2.01	Lambert, Morton et al. (2004); Burlingame et al. (2005)	Adults & youth	https://www.oqmeasures.com/
Partners for Change Outcome Management System (PCOMS ORS and SRS)	Miller et al. (2005); Miller et al. (2003); Duncan et al. (2003); Duncan & Reese (2015)	Adults & youth	https://betteroutcomesnow.com/about-bon/ https://www.scottdmiller.com/
Patient Case Management Information System (PCMIS; PHQ-9/GAD-7)	Delgadillo et al. (2018)	Adults	https://www.york.ac.uk/healthsciences/pc-mis/
NORSE	Moltu et al. (2021)	Adults	https://www.norsefeedback.no/en/
Treatment Outcome Package (TOP)	Kraus et al. (2005)	Adults	http://www.outcomereferrals.com/main/sub-page/category/top-assessment/top-assessment

I started with progress feedback doing it with paper and pencil as a young therapist working with youth. Then, when I became a clinic director, I found myself thinking about some sticky questions like 'How do I keep my referral streams going?', 'How do I know who to assign to what therapist?', 'How do I know how treatment is going with my therapists, aside from weekly supervision?, and 'How do I hear the patient's voice in all of this, so that it doesn't get filtered by the therapist?'. So, we just made a feedback system using excel spreadsheets. It is helpful not thinking of feedback as collecting data or having a metric, but as a way of visualizing progress, so that the therapist and the patient can both see it and have a shared understanding.
 – Susan Douglas, feedback coach and implementation researcher, USA

Conclusions

We have set out the key issues in deciding on a measure and practical issues that need to be considered when choosing an outcome measure. Given that the focus of this text is on providing and guiding therapists with the information as to *how* to select a measure, we have explicitly not made any recommendations or given favour to one measure over another. That is, we have explicitly eschewed both going into detail about measures and also in advising any one existing measure over another. It is likely that new measures will become available and the principles and procedures contained in this chapter should be equally applicable to such measures.

Key points of this chapter

- Monitoring and feedback during the course of treatment have clear advantages over the simple measurement of outcomes before and after treatment.
- Key considerations in selecting an outcome instrument include its length, relevance and accessibility, psychometric properties, sensitivity to change, and costs.
- In most typical outpatient psychological therapies settings, a measure with a weekly timeframe likely works best for monitoring and feedback.
- The measurement frequency should be tailored to the patient population. In treatments up to 20 sessions, session-by-session measurements are optimal; in longer treatments, less frequent measurements might be more sustainable.
- Measuring just before the start of each session is usually optimal.
- The mode of administration may determine the type of feedback that can be used and should be tailored to the size and budget of the service.

3 Barriers and enablers for implementation

In this chapter

Despite the known benefits of routine outcome monitoring in supporting the development of practice-based evidence and improving clinical outcomes, it is well known that achieving a successful implementation of measurement in routine care is highly challenging. Several authors have previously discussed barriers to the adoption and effective use of routine outcome measurement and feedback. Studies have shown that feedback effects are dependent on implementation issues, such as therapist behaviour, attitudes, application, and commitment to feedback. Therefore, simply establishing a routine of measurement in a treatment system does not guarantee improved results. Successful implementation requires a detailed understanding of barriers and enablers, which are commonly grouped according to broad themes, such as organizational, technological, practical, attitudinal, and competency-related barriers. Such barriers are summarized in this chapter, along with well-documented enablers that support successful implementation.

Preparing to implement a ROM system at an organizational level

As stated earlier, in principle, any outcome measure can be used to measure, monitor, or provide feedback but practicalities will have a major impact on the decision-making process. So, it may be that you or your service is familiar with using a particular outcome measure in providing summary information on patient outcomes at the start and end of therapy. The decision then becomes whether to build a more developed monitoring and feedback system around the existing measure(s) or to adopt a different outcome measure that is associated with feedback procedures. Regardless of that specific decision, extending administration to a repeated or sessional basis needs to be carried out with the backing of therapists. Accordingly, we set out some guidance on how to make this stepped change in the use of ROM and feedback.

Openly discussing hopes and fears

The reasons for the implementation and expectations for staff and for the service should be clear and explicit from the start of any implementation project. The reasons should be focused on enhancing the quality of the service for patients rather than on any form of performance management of therapists. However, a fundamental component is to recognize that implementing a feedback system into any health care system is an organizational intervention. It will affect most, if not all, aspects of the working environment for therapists, patients, and managers and, as such, the success or otherwise of implementing any system lies in the preparatory work carried out prior to implementation, primarily with the therapists whereby the hopes and fears regarding such a system are discussed openly. This key process sounds simple, but it is all too often overlooked.

The main aim of such a process is to openly discuss concerns and aspirations. It should therefore involve all therapists and associated team members, particularly administrative staff – in fact, anyone for whom the new system will have an impact. The process involves enabling people to openly voice their concerns, as one of the key reasons why any implementation of such a system fails is that the implementation could stumble at multiple hurdles. Some hopes, when discussed openly, will be found to be unrealistic, and so will some fears. Such fears may include feeling that therapists will be performance-managed according to their patient outcomes, or that it will fuel a competitive climate between therapists if their performance data is openly shared. They may become overly focused on concerns as to whether the data will show them not to be as effective as they thought they were. Such a view might then make a practitioner feel that they have to be more selective with their patients and only take on those for whom they consider have the best chance of achieving a good outcome. Others will be concerned that it will involve more administrative work, taking up valuable time or that there will be no time allowance for such tasks. The key point here is that when the private hopes and fears are openly shared they can then be addressed. In turn, this dialogue offers an opportunity to emphasize the aspects of ROM and feedback that hold most value for therapists: having a structured and measurable way to assess progress continuously, having more information to inform the treatment plan, having a valuable data source to learn about what works in therapy, having a mechanism to evaluate one's practice, and to form a professional development plan that could help to improve effectiveness.

Champions and early adopters

As with the hopes and fears exercise, a key aim is to develop a *process* of implementation. In any implementation, it will usually work best if it is not carried out all at once. So, implementation could start with those therapists who are enthusiastic to try it – *champions*. It is invariably the case that within any group of therapists there is either someone or a few people who are more likely and prepared to adopt a monitoring or feedback system. Having so-called champions within a team provides a key way forward in enabling other therapists to see that this need not be a staff versus management issue. Similarly, if the service comprises various teams, it might be that one of these teams might be an *early adopter* for the implementation and support each other, feeding back to other therapists. In our experience, close partnership with early adopters is essential for effective implementation, and this works best when the early adopters have credibility and influence among their peers. In many domains of human activity, some people exert an influence on others who mimic their behaviour, because they are seen as role models or good exemplars of that particular domain of activity. Identifying the *influencers* within an organization or clinical team and maximizing their interest and motivation to be an early adopter is a good strategy for implementation. In our work, we have partnered up with therapists who were seen to be opinion leaders in their team, and we ensured that we understood and fulfilled their incentives to become involved in an implementation project. For, example, some of these clinical influencers eventually became co-authors of our published work; they became clinical supervisors or organizers of feedback-focused practice development groups, etc.

> *If you roll it out in the future, using people like me who find it really helpful might encourage others to do it.*
> – Anonymous therapist, UK

Pilot stage and stepped wedge rollout

In moving beyond the initial stages of implementation, a key stage comes in rolling out the system at all levels of a service. A suggested programme would comprise initially setting out the rollout as a pilot project for a specified period of time, with one team or group of the service responding to being identified as an early adopter. Such a model is more likely to be accepted and it also provides the opportunity to evaluate its success in terms of issues raised during the pilot period. Following an evaluation, it can then be decided on how to proceed and, if so, what might be improved for the implementation to run smoothly. We highly advise to include patients in the evaluation process, to assess to what extent the ROM tool is acceptable to them. Thereafter, in any rollout, there is merit in adopting what is often referred to as a *stepped wedge design* in which the system is rolled out over a period of time, introducing new teams at intervals whereby they can adjust and improve aspects of the implementation in light of prior experience. Such a strategy also makes the whole process more manageable and means that resources, which are likely to be limited, can be focused on one team or group of people at a time. This will also allow any bespoke adaptations if necessary.

One key message arising from the procedures outlined here is that implementing any system of monitoring or feedback takes time and the critical component is to ensure that all those involved are onboard. The above steps of implementation can be hampered by a number of barriers, and therefore the next section covers the most common barriers and potential solutions.

The key stakeholder in ROM and feedback is the patient. Start your conversations about implementation with them. It is their data. They are interested in their progress. We have found that lesson again and again. Every time I listen to that advice, we are able to get to creative solutions faster than if we start with what we, the researchers and clinical staff think is best.

– Andrew Page, feedback researcher, Australia

Developing a narrative

Progress feedback as an intervention is not specifically linked to one treatment orientation, but can rather be seen as a generic intervention that can be used in treatments of all orientations. From an implementation perspective, feedback will be more likely to stick if therapists can really make it their own and can find a way to integrate it into their therapies. And of course, when feedback is more fully integrated into the therapy provided, patients will also be more motivated and the information that is being collected will have more intrinsic value for both the patient and the therapist. In our experience, some therapists find it easy to fit progress feedback into their way of working, whereas others either see it as something that is happening outside of their therapy, or experience it as something that interferes with their way of working.

We regularly give talks on ROM and feedback at therapist conferences and after one such talk a psychodynamic therapist asked, 'Do you know if there is any research on how ROM ruins the therapeutic alliance? Because it does!'. This therapist clearly had not been able to integrate ROM into their way of working yet. When talking to therapists who had been able to integrate ROM and feedback into their way of working – and they can be found in all treatment orientations – what we have noticed is that they seemed to have created a narrative for themselves that made ROM and feedback fit in with their treatment orientation. From that narrative, they could also communicate with their patients on the usefulness of ROM and feedback for the treatment. For this book, we have interviewed therapists from different orientations and asked them how they integrated working with feedback with their general way of working as a therapist. Below you can find some of their responses.

In a humanistic approach to therapy, one of the early goals of treatment is to become fellow humans with different roles in an addressing a problem. So, using feedback to establish a third position or an object outside the dyad, is helpful to that. And also, when you work experientially, then you're very much working in the here and now with the client, often working with emotional processes in detail. And then, in my view, you could easily miss part of the story. So, ROM and feedback is an extra chance for the patient to provide me with information. A full narrative of how they are doing in life, so that we're not losing track of the whole, while focusing on these specific details that we're working on."

– Christian Moltu, emotion-focused therapist and feedback researcher, Norway

I think one of the things that characterizes the role of the therapist in CBT is that we consider ourselves to be equals with our clients. I bring my expertise; the client brings theirs. They are the expert about their own life and personality, I have learned things in school that might be helpful, and together we can try to figure things out. And I think what really helps with ROM for me is that it actively puts responsibility on the clients to voice their own concerns. They're automatically part of the therapy. They have a part to do that is explicit. This is your way of letting me know how you're doing. I mean, of course you can tell me, but this is how we can check and keep track of it.
— Kim de Jong, feedback researcher and CBT therapist,
the Netherlands

To me, ROM and feedback is an intervention you do in the relationship. Especially when we are talking about the alliance feedback that some ROM systems provide. When you ask someone to give you feedback, you ask specifically for negative feedback and encourage that. It's very anxiety provoking and it's very well suited to kind of trigger all kinds of defence mechanisms in the client, that you can see. And that is kind of food for the therapy. You know, and then, when the client chooses to go out on a limb and do something that they are not usually doing in their relationships [give negative feedback, ed.], and the therapist can respond in a different way than the patient expects, you can provide a corrective emotional experience. So, to me, it really is an intervention.
— Heidi Brattland, integrative/psychodynamic therapist
and feedback researcher, Norway

For me it is easy, because ROM and feedback fits in a scientific way of working. I use scientifically-based methods and use a scientific language and also work explicitly with hypothesis-testing in my treatment. Then it is important that you also look at the results of the therapy: is there any progress? Does this method fit? Are we doing the right thing? I assume that every licensed psychologist does that.
— Erik van der Put, cognitive behavioural therapist,
the Netherlands

In family therapy, there is the notion that every system has the capacity to adjust to a healthier way of coping when information on for instance each family member's perception and relation to others is shared. Because couple and family therapy is more complex than individual therapy with respect to the amount of information when more than one client is present, ROM is experienced as a tool that enables me to organize this information in a user-friendly and rational way. The sharing of ROM information within the couple- or family system has thus in itself the potential power to create the needed and desired changes, thereby representing a vital change mechanism with respect to therapy process and outcome.
— Terje Tilden, feedback researcher and family therapist, Norway

Barriers to successful implementation of ROM and feedback

Organizational barriers

Organizational barriers refer to aspects of a service's policies, resources, culture or incentives, which make it difficult to implement routine outcome monitoring. For example, services where therapists have high caseloads may struggle to implement ROM due to a lack of time in between therapy appointments to administer, score, and interpret measures. Having additional time in between appointments and resources to overcome time constraints can help in this regard, such as support from an administrator that can issue paper-and-pen questionnaires at a clinic reception, or an electronic system that can send (via mobile text or email), collect, and score measures efficiently. Even in an optimal situation where the therapist has access to a computer in the clinic room, has an automated data collection system, and has time in between therapy sessions to evaluate this information, cultural aspects of the organization may pose obstacles. For example, routine outcome measurement may not be expected as part of service policies, in which case therapists may have little incentive to do this routinely, since it is an effortful task. On the other hand, decision-makers in an organization that requires outcome measurement as part of service policy might use this in a way that could be perceived as potentially punitive (i.e., if attaining poor outcomes could carry risks for the therapist's salary, reputation, or relationships with supervisors and peers). Some organizations might use outcome measurement primarily for reporting purposes, to satisfy their funders or stakeholders, rather than as a decision-support strategy that can benefit patients' quality of care and therapists' professional development. Such a culture could potentially undermine the therapists' commitment to and effective use of outcome measures, simply treating this as a 'box-ticking' exercise rather than a process that is integral to evidence-based psychological care. In contexts where services work towards specific performance targets (i.e., specified by funders, stakeholders, or regulators), perverse incentives can arise, which can raise obstacles to effective and ethical use of routine outcome monitoring. For example, the imposition of performance targets can put clinical services in a position where they may feel compelled to be overly selective of patients who they deem most 'suitable' or likely to benefit from therapy, thus limiting access to care for those who perhaps have more severe and complicated problems. In these situations, outcome measures could be unethically used to restrict access to care for people with high symptom severity, or data might be selectively collected/reported for patients who respond well to treatment.

As illustrated in the above examples, there are a number of organizational barriers that can make it difficult to adopt ROM in an ethical and effective way. As such, at an organizational level, services seeking to implement and support the use of ROM effectively could consider the following questions as a general checklist of issues to address.

Policies and incentives

• Do therapists have basic training in psychometrics and outcome measurement practices? If not, is training available to them as part of their job?
• Does the organization have a policy on which measures are appropriate to apply with the target clinical population?
• Does the service have a policy on the frequency and method of routine outcome monitoring, in a way that fully integrates it into the therapy process for each patient?
• Do therapists have sufficient time to administer, score, interpret, and integrate measures into their clinical practice?
• Are therapists expected to discuss measures with their patients and with their supervisors as part of service policy?
• Is outcome measurement clearly integrated into the service's clinical supervision and practice development processes?
• Could some organizational policies potentially introduce perverse incentives that undermine the effective or ethical use of measurement? How could the service strive to mitigate the influence of perverse incentives?

Resources

• Do therapists have access to validated questionnaires, scoring, and interpretation rules?
• Do therapists have administrative support or technology that can enable the efficient collection of measures?
• Does the service have access to computerized outcome monitoring and feedback technologies?
• Do therapists have access to computer technology in their clinic rooms to facilitate the real-time use of feedback technologies?
• In the absence of computer technologies in the clinic room, do therapists have access to photocopied charts or other materials that can support paper-and-pen outcome monitoring?

Culture

• Are decision-makers and clinical leaders supportive of outcome measurement? If not, what are their concerns? How can such concerns be addressed?
• Is there someone in the organization with responsibility for overseeing and monitoring the implementation and effective use of measurement? Does this person have the expertise, time, and resources to support implementation?
• Is measurement integrated into clinical case discussions, clinical supervision, and professional development plans?

- Does the organization take a punitive stance towards outcome measurement and performance targets? If yes, this could be an obstacle to effective and ethical use of measurement, in which case clinical leaders could undertake a consultation with their employees to better understand their perspectives, attitudes, and concerns. A process of consultation could help to co-produce a set of expectations and procedures that are acceptable to therapists and patients, and which value their professional growth and development.

To some extent, the organizational pressures that make implementation of outcome measurement challenging have some relation to the old adage: '*good, fast, and cheap: you can choose two but you can't have all three*'. The successful implementation of routine outcome monitoring and feedback in a way that is 'good' (i.e., clinically effective) and 'fast' (i.e., rapid adoption at a service-wide level) is certainly not 'cheap'. Successful implementation is expensive, because it requires resources/technology, time, training, consultation, and continual evaluation. Aiming for a less expensive implementation necessarily involves cutting some corners and making some compromises. For instance, deciding not to invest in an industry-standard data collection and feedback system may be a 'cheap' option, but it may not be as 'good'. Similarly, reducing the cost necessary to allow therapists to have sufficient administrative time in between therapy appointments might be a 'cheap' option, but not as 'good'. Implementing routine outcome monitoring by making it a mandatory aspect of practice could lead to 'fast' adoption by all therapists and supervisors, but neglecting to invest the time and cost necessary to train staff to properly understand and integrate measures into their practice may not lead to 'good' results. On the other hand, an implementation plan that attends to and invests in all relevant costs can lead to 'good' results, but the full and proper integration may not be 'fast', since it takes time to consult with stakeholders, to align services policies to support the goals of outcome monitoring, to train staff, to embed measurement into the organizational audit, and service improvement cycle, etc.

> *In order to implement measurement, actually the first thing that you have got to do is to identify the problems. Allow therapists to identify what are the challenges and how, as a service, to overcome those challenges.*
> – John Mellor-Clark, implementation expert and feedback system developer, UK

Technological barriers

Technological barriers concern the materials and systems used to collect, store, and process outcomes data. Three levels of technological barriers are relevant to implementation. At a basic level, the selection of measures chosen for a particular patient or clinical sample can in itself limit implementation, if such a selection is overly burdensome (i.e., too lengthy), or lacks face validity to the intended user (i.e., it doesn't make sense to the patient). A burdensome or inadequate set of measures can thus undermine the completeness and validity of clinical data, even if the service has access to modern electronic surveys or computerized technologies to collect and process data. At an intermediate level, we can think of data collection and storage technologies. Of course, therapists can simply collect paper-and-pen questionnaires and store these in written or printed notes, or tabulate them using spreadsheets. However, computerized data collection systems can enable a more efficient way to collect, search, and evaluate data in a systematic way, since this enables multiple therapists to contribute to a structured archive of clinical data. Thus, a barrier at this intermediate level of data collection would be the lack of a structured data management system or software. At the more advanced level, clinical services may already have an appropriate set of measures that are collected in a systematic way using an industry-standard data management system. However, large-volume clinical data are difficult to process and use in a way that is directly relevant to individual therapy cases. Some computerized feedback systems process data and provide automated feedback to therapists, based on clinical data from large clinical samples (as described in Chapter 1). Such systems are particularly designed to support clinical practice by enabling therapists to assess their patients' treatment response with greater accuracy, particularly enabling them to identify patients at risk of poor treatment response in a timely way. Thus, a barrier for services that already use modern data collection systems may be the lack of availability of processing technologies such as expected treatment response (ETR) curves or other feedback signalling tools described in Chapter 1. There are a number of ways to maximize the use of technology and to remove related barriers:

• Select measures that are brief, easy to complete and which are closely matched to the target clinical population.
• As far as possible, automate the collection of data by using email or modern technologies such as mobile text messages with embedded weblinks to electronic surveys that can be completed easily using a smartphone.
• At a service-wide level, adopt the use of industry-standard data management systems, rather than traditional paper-pen archiving or spreadsheets.
• Consider adopting available feedback systems that use state-of-the-art signalling technologies (i.e., expected treatment response curves or other prediction algorithms). Alternatively, consider working with academic researchers who can help to develop such technologies using routinely collected outcomes data.

Practical barriers

Practical barriers include inadequate planning, procedures, or resources to adequately adopt routine outcome monitoring. To some extent, such barriers have some relation to wider organizational or financial constraints. Some examples of practical barriers are:

- Not having access to a photocopier, or a set of printed questionnaires ahead of time.
- Not having a computer available in the clinic room to display outcome monitoring or feedback graphs.
- Therapy sessions scheduled in a way that prevents the consistent collection or review of outcome measures.
- Such barriers tend to be more evident in the early stages of adoption of routine outcome monitoring and can be overcome as therapists gain experience in this process and are able to request and access the necessary resources. Although these types of barriers may seem obvious, it can be useful to try to anticipate such practical barriers ahead of time and as part of an implementation plan, for instance by consulting with therapists during the early stages of project planning.

Attitudinal barriers

Attitudinal barriers and resistance to the use of outcome measurement can arise in different groups of stakeholders, including managers, therapists, and patients. If the use of data is not seen as a priority by managers, and if an organization lacks systems to incentivize its application (e.g., as part of clinical supervision), therapists are less likely to effectively implement it. Similarly, patients can sometimes resist or forget to regularly complete outcome measures for a variety of reasons. Chapter 4 in this book extensively covers common attitudinal problems that arise in therapists and patients, so we refer the reader to that section, which also covers several recommended solutions and strategies to enable implementation.

Competency-related barriers

Competency-related barriers can be seen as deficits in knowledge and skills that support the effective use of outcome measures. In our experience, therapists are less likely to adopt routine outcome monitoring in their practice without a thorough understanding of the following questions:

- Why should we use outcome measures in psychological practice? (See Chapter 1)
- Which measures should I use? (See Chapter 2)
- How do I explain the purpose and rationale for outcome measurement to my patients? (See Chapter 5)
- How do I interpret these measures clinically? (See Chapter 6)
- How do I support patients to adhere to routine outcome monitoring? (See Chapter 6)
- What do I do if my patient is not responding well to treatment according to the measures? (See Chapters 7–8)

Competency-related barriers can be overcome by a combination of formal training, self-directed reading of case examples, and instructional guidelines, and guided practice (i.e., observed by or in consultation with a supervisor or peer). To a large extent, the purpose of this book is to provide practical guidelines to overcome competency-related barriers. As such, we refer readers and educators to the above questions and related chapters of the book, as a general blueprint to develop competence in the systematic use of routine outcome monitoring.

This may sound heretical, but I am less interested in measurement than I ever have been, I am so much more interested in the use of this information to support patient-centred communication. To create that shared understanding when your patients can look at a graph or be able to say: 'Oh my gosh, that is when this event happened, and you can see how I was feeling'. That does so much for the therapeutic alliance, that ability to surface what is important to your patient and not have it filtered by the therapist first. I think of measurement progress feedback as a truly an empowerment tool in the right hands.
– Susan Douglas, feedback coach and implementation researcher, USA

Necessary support system and resources

Leadership and management

It is important at the outset to view the implementation of ROM and clinical feedback as an organizational intervention. As such, there needs to be clear leadership and management in place that is effective. In a small clinic or organization these roles may be filled by the same person; in larger organizations, by different people. Whatever the set-up is, there needs to be clarity as to the roles and responsibilities. The leadership role needs to have the authority to make decisions on behalf of the team and the management of the implementation needs to be at the operational level. These two roles should be distinguished from that of therapists who might act as champions for ROM and clinical feedback: leadership and management roles carry organizational responsibilities; being a champion requires enthusiasm for the implementation and use of ROM.

Contextual climate

While leadership and management are crucial, there needs to be a consensus within the clinic or organization to work with the initiative. However, achieving such consensus requires a process that needs the involvement of all staff if implementation is to be successful. This process requires addressing the *hopes and fears* of therapists which is described earlier in this chapter.

Administration

For any system of measurement to be informative, there needs to be an infrastructure that supports its implementation, processing, and providing output at the time it is needed. This aspect can all-too-often be forgotten or only considered late in the planning stage. However, without the necessary support, all good efforts to address the previous points will fall flat if there is insufficient infrastructure. The two key elements are invariably human (i.e., people to support the programme) and information technology (IT) and both can work from a basic model (single person working with a spreadsheet) to a fully-funded team utilizing purchased software packages for data collection and analyses. It is likely that implementation will be more successful if a single IT system is used – that is, the practitioner does not have to utilize multiple electronic systems. Nevertheless, as explained in Chapter 2, there are different models of administration: no-tech, lo-tech and high-tech methods. The choice of method for a particular service often requires considerations about cost and budget.

Financial support

While outcome measurement only requires two administrations, outcome monitoring will require considerably more. Hence, if a proprietary measure is used, changing to a monitoring system will have considerable cost implications. We therefore recommend cost-neutral measures – that is, measures that are either in the public domain, copy left, or under Creative Commons License. Some measures may require a registration but then incurs no cost; it is simply a form of capturing the potential use of a measure by measure developers.

Timescale

The final component is to set a timeline for training and implementation. It is often thought that the decision making and particularly the implementation period can be achieved relatively quickly. However, unless a realistic timeframe is set, implementation is less likely to be successful.

Implementation science and policy drivers for adoption

In view of the multiple barriers to implementation, consensus in the field is that multiple strategies tailored to address locally relevant obstacles are necessary for successful implementation. Strategies drawn from implementation science (e.g., Lewis et al., 2019; Nilsen, 2020) have been described by several authors. For example, Mellor-Clark et al. (2016) recommend creating a pre-implementation plan and service profile survey, listing known and expected obstacles and enablers (described above). It is also known that formal training that addresses known attitudinal and competency-related barriers can be a successful way to promote adoption of new technologies and processes in health care (e.g., Casper et al., 2007).

Drawing from these sources and case examples, organizations that plan to implement routine outcome monitoring in clinical care should:

- Nominate an implementation leader, supported by an implementation team.
- The team should carry out consultations and/or surveys with key stakeholders, specifically aiming to map out potential barriers and to generate proposed solutions.
- Careful attention and planning should go into the three levels of technological enablers: (1) which measures? (2) which data collection system will enable standardisation? and (3) how can modern feedback signalling tools be adopted?
- An implementation plan should fully cost all aspects of implementation including technology, resources and clinical time necessary to train therapists and to enable them sufficient administrative time in daily practice to effectively integrate this into their work.
- Policies should be aligned to support outcome monitoring as an integral aspect of therapy, clinical supervision, and practice development.
- The organization should adopt a minimum standard of training concerning outcome measurement for new employees, ideally recruiting new staff with the expected competencies, but also embedding training and development on these competencies as part of practice development activities for existing staff. Ongoing development can be achieved through formal training workshops, directed reading, clinical case discussions, and interest groups that meet to share case studies and good practice in ROM and feedback.
- The implementation team should monitor the progress of adoption in routine care, with reference to specific milestones and indicators of success (i.e., time-specific data completeness targets, evidence of adoption into clinical case notes, supervision records and annual professional development reviews).

From a wider healthcare system perspective, the American Psychological Association (APA) *Mental and Behavioral Health Registry Initiative* proposed six key recommendations to enable psychological services to adopt routine outcome monitoring (Wright et al., 2020):

- Patient-reported outcome measures should be central to ensure person-centred care.
- Measures that are relevant across a wide group of individuals receiving care should be prioritized.
- These measures should have rigorously established psychometric properties.
- These measures should be used to support continuous quality improvement initiatives in line with the principles of a learning health system.
- Implementation should be supported by high-quality training.
- Regulatory and professional bodies should lead the development of measures and the establishment of training standards for practising psychologists.

Advice from the experts

During the process of writing this book, we have interviewed several experts in the field of ROM and feedback, and we have asked them the question: if someone would ask you, 'Where do I start with the implementation of feedback?' what would you reply? Here are their answers:

We were so naive when we started the implementation of feedback. A colleague had gone to a workshop and came back very enthusiastic, and we decided to implement it into our service. We knew nothing about feedback or implementation. It took so much time and effort. Over time, we became more effective in the way we were training people, in how we introduced it to patients. My advice? Before you start, talk to people with experience in feedback implementation, in any system, as the principles of the implementation are alike for all feedback systems."
– Heidi Brattland, feedback researcher and therapist, Norway

"Start by asking yourself questions like "what is our current culture of data-informed decision making?", "How is the psychological safety in our teams?" and "How confident do people feel about using feedback in treatment?" And then use the answers to those questions to help align working with feedback with the way we work on a day-to-day basis. Think about how you can build the strongest foundation first, and build your feedback system on top of that.
– Susan Douglas, feedback coach and implementation researcher, USA

Any outcome instrument will likely show that you help about half of your patients improve reliably. As a service, you need to ask yourself: am I comfortable with that 50% or do I want to know about the 50% that I am not helping? Because those are your teachers. They are going to help you understand how you can help more people.
– John Mellor-Clark, implementation expert and feedback system developer, UK

Remember that the idea of feedback is simple. And yet there are all these complexities around implementation. Those complexities are real and we need to grapple with them, but as we grapple with the complexities, we can anchor ourselves in that this is a very simple idea, that we are trying to implement.
– Andrew Page, feedback researcher and therapist, Australia

We were teaching people how to use the measures and not how to implement a feedback culture in their work. Culture of feedback is the biggest topic. So, we're starting to talk about creating an atmosphere where the client has the space to speak up. Most importantly about things that the client might deem too small to complain about. We want them to openly discuss their experience. Open their minds. Let us hear all of the thoughts, positive and negative, about us, as the process unfolds. So, I would say that the key concept is how to create that culture in routine outcome monitoring.
– Scott Miller, feedback system developer and trainer, USA

Are you prepared for this to be a long process? The rewards will be there, but it will not happen overnight, you can expect it to take 5–8 years. And it is really not about the measures, it is about culture change, it is about thinking differently about our cases, about thinking differently about outcomes and being open to the fact that we may need to shift the way that we do things.
 – Robbie Babins-Wagner, counselling centre CEO, Canada

Give therapists time to learn this and accept this new way of working. Help them make use of the feedback in their clinical decisions. That is a big part of implementation. Now, we have video training and other resources therapists can use when the treatment is not progressing. We just try to help therapists make better use of the information coming out of feedback systems.
 – Wolfgang Lutz, feedback researcher and therapist, Germany

It was necessary for us to build in a feedback loop into the system development and that feedback loop was continuous, meaning that we will always strive through new iterations to get closer and closer to the clinical concepts that we aim to measure. Patients and therapists differ in their needs for changes in the system. A patient has expert experience with their particular problem or process, and many of them will put in requests for more specificity. Therapists are more conceptual in their feedback on the system and comment on what they want the feedback system to cover that it currently does not cover well.
 – Christian Moltu, feedback system developer, researcher, and therapist, Norway

In Box 3.1, we discuss an example of a very successful implementation of routine outcome monitoring and feedback in the Calgary Counselling Centre. The Calgary Counselling Centre is a charitable organization that has been offering psychological interventions for people with common mental health problems since 1962. They support individuals and families with a dedicated team of mental health professionals and volunteers. Guided by a bold vision to become a centre of excellence in psychological practice and research, this organization has embedded outcome measurement in routine care and leveraged practice-based data to establish a cycle of learning and improvement over several years.

Box 3.1 A case example of successful ROM implementation

Having a mature and effective implementation of ROM in routine care took a considerable amount of effort and time. This effort was led by *Dr Robbie Babins-Wagner*, a visionary leader in the field of ROM, through a four-phase process that started around the year 2000.

Phase 1: Selecting the feedback instruments

The first phase involved a consultation with leaders and staff at the centre to communicate the rationale of ROM and to obtain support from key stakeholders. A key question during this phase was to decide which outcome measure to use. Using a democratic process, counsellors had the opportunity to pilot the use of one measure during six months, and then to pilot a different measure during another six months, after which they voted to decide their preferred measure. At the end of this phase, a choice was made for a measure of psychological distress (OQ-45) prior to every session and a measure of the treatment process (Session Rating Scale) at the end of each session.

Phase 2: Implementation into routine care

This process enabled an important step towards implementation in the second phase between 2004 and 2008. Towards the end of that time period, an analysis of routinely collected data revealed that the ROM process was only being implemented with around 40 per cent of patients.

Phase 3: Creating a learning culture

This observation led to the third phase 2008–2011, where the centre adopted a policy of mandatory data collection. Importantly, this policy prioritized the need to collect ROM data, but did not tie the clinical outcomes or results of the measures into performance reviews for counsellors. This policy balances the goal of creating a learning health system without imposing the burden of 'payment by results' on counsellors, which could have adverse consequences on staff morale and could adversely affect data accuracy. In addition, during this phase the centre employed an external consultant with expertise in the use of ROM and feedback, which served as an incentive and source of support to guide counsellors on how to maximise the use of measures.

Phase 4: Data-driven improvement

From 2011 onwards, the fourth phase was characterized by a gradual culture change in the organization. Initially, counsellors started to receive, discuss, and reflect on centre-wide reports on clinical outcomes. The learning from this process eventually supported counsellors to be open to receiving and reviewing their own outcome reports, which in turn provided useful data for their practice development and supervision consultations. With the growth of practice-based data, the centre began to produce important contributions to psychotherapy research. For example, two seminal studies used data from this organization to investigate if clinical supervisors influence the variability in patients' clinical outcomes (Rousmaniere et al., 2016) and whether or not counsellors' clinical outcomes improve over time (Goldberg et al., 2016a). Another study reports that year-on-year improvements in patient outcomes over the course of time were achieved at this centre through a combination of progress feedback and a forum where counsellors discuss difficult cases (Goldberg et al., 2016b). The title of this study truly captures the essence of what the Calgary Counselling Centre has achieved over time through their remarkable commitment to practice-based evidence, 'Creating a climate for therapist improvement'.

Conclusions

The effectiveness of ROM and feedback is largely dependent on the extent to which it is embedded into the clinical routine of therapists and services. Like any innovation in health care, the successful adoption of ROM requires a comprehensive implementation strategy. This implementation strategy should have teamwork and participatory decision-making at its core, and it should be designed in such a way that expected barriers can be pre-empted and matched with known strategies to overcome these difficulties.

Key points in this chapter

* Successful implementation of ROM in health care services usually involves: (1) preparatory tasks to introduce measurement to staff; (2) organization of an implementation team; (3) mapping of potential barriers and enablers; (4) a pilot phase; (5) a full implementation phase; and (6) the establishment of a data-informed learning culture.

* Involving therapists and wider support staff in open dialogue about their hopes and fears can help to understand and pre-empt potential roadblocks to implementation.

* There are multiple barriers (organizational, practical, attitudinal, competence-related) to implementation and matched strategies to remove or work around these barriers.

* There are many examples of successful implementation across various countries, and experts in the field converge in the observation that successful implementation requires committed leadership, teamwork, resources, and time to move from idea to full adoption.

4 Common problems and solutions to promote adherence to routine outcome monitoring

In this chapter

So far, we have explained how to introduce, administer and implement outcome measures into routine clinical practice in cases with minimal obstacles to this. In practice, however, several issues can arise, which make this process difficult. Here, we outline some common difficulties and suggested strategies to deal with this. These difficulties are organized according to issues that are related to the therapist and issues that are related to the patient. We recognize that not all of these obstacles may be relevant to readers who are experienced ROM and feedback users. For this reason, in this chapter we refer to therapists in the third person, in the understanding that they may recognize some of these difficulties in their own practice or in the practice of others (i.e., supervisees or students).

Therapist difficulties

Uncertainty about measure selection

A common obstacle to feedback-informed treatment is the therapist's uncertainty about which measure to select and apply in routine care. Hesitation in the selection of measures can lead to delays in the proper implementation of routine outcome monitoring, missing the valuable information that is collected in a baseline (pre-treatment measure) and the earliest stages of treatment. In Chapter 3, we have outlined principles of good practice in the selection of outcome measures, such as attention to measures that are:

* matched to the patient's problems and goals
* valid, reliable and with established psychometric norms
* accessible – brief, easy, translated if necessary
* affordable or free to use.

In order to minimize uncertainty and loss of valuable information, it is a good idea to use a multi-domain strategy for outcome monitoring, including one general measure of distress or functioning (see examples of measures in Chapter 2) and one additional measure that may be specifically matched to the person's presenting problems as defined diagnostically or through a collaborative formulation of the main presenting problems (at an initial assessment). In this way, the general measure of distress can be applied from the very start and can be supplemented with more specific measures that best align to key problems. For example, the Outcome Questionnaire (OQ-45; Lambert et al., 2004) or the Clinical Outcomes in Routine Evaluation (e.g., CORE-OM; Barkham et al., 2010) could be selected as a general measure of distress, each of which has well-established population norms, psychometric properties and interpretation rules (i.e., reliable change index and clinical cut-off). Such a measure could then be supplemented with a symptom-specific measure for patients with specific problems such as post-traumatic stress disorder, obsessive-compulsive disorder, social anxiety disorder, etc. This uncertainty about measure selection tends to be a matter of greater concern in private practice or in services that treat highly heterogeneous patient populations, whereas it tends to be less problematic in services that treat more homogeneous patient groups with similar presenting problems – in which case the adoption of a standard battery of measures is appropriate.

The Holy Grail fallacy

Uncertainty about measure selection is closely related to another problem – *the Holy Grail fallacy*, which is the belief that there must be a measure that perfectly captures the symptoms, problems and goals that are most relevant to each patient. A common experience when therapists are considering different questionnaires is that they disagree with the wording, content, length or structure of the questionnaires under consideration. Therapists often find that available measures do not adequately reflect their patients' key concerns, or the processes that the therapist expects to be relevant to that patient's progress in therapy. Therapists often feel like they either need to modify the available questionnaires somehow, or combine multiple questionnaires, or construct new questionnaires altogether. All of these are common indicators of the Holy Grail fallacy.

Unless the therapist is a trained and experienced psychometrician, modifying validated questionnaires or developing new ones is not advisable. Research in the field has documented over 100 different patient-reported outcome measures, many with established validity and reliability (Wahl et al., 2010). To some extent, the large volume and diversity of measures illustrates the problem in question: theorists, therapists and psychometricians continue to develop numerous patient-reported measures in search of the Holy Grail. Ironically, many of the well-validated questionnaires are significantly correlated, which indicates that they may well be measuring the same or highly similar underlying constructs and aspects of psychological distress (Batterham et al., 2018). The fact that commonly used measures of psychological distress can actually be mapped onto one another (i.e., a score in one scale can be translated into the relevant scale of another correlated measure) illustrates the superfluous nature of the Holy Grail fallacy. On this basis, we recommend taking a pragmatic approach by selecting a small set of 'good enough' measures following the selection principles outlined in the previous section.

> *Implementation is a process of mutual maturation. People get to experience, understand, and live from their own perspective and so that is how they approach comments about the feedback system as well. We try to make something that works well across the board, and some suggestions for improvement can be realized and others cannot. As long as that conversation is ongoing and all parties feel that it is constructive. But obviously the user will need to deal with some disappointment in that. No system can be perfect. But I think throughout the process, it is easier to accept that when you understand why and how and what the trade-offs are.*
> – Christian Moltu, Feedback system developer and researcher, Norway

The omniscience fallacy

Therapists that altogether refuse to use routine outcome monitoring, and those who use it ineffectively, are sometimes influenced by *the omniscience fallacy*, which is the belief that clinical judgement is the most trustworthy source of information about the patient's problems and treatment response. Therapists that adopt this line of reasoning often dismiss outcome measures altogether, or use them in an inconsistent way, selectively attending to results that confirm their clinical intuition and ignoring the results that don't fit.

The omniscience fallacy has a long history in the fields of psychiatry and psychotherapy. Diagnostic manuals such as the DSM-V reify clinical judgement as central to the psychiatric assessment process, guiding therapists to 'trust' their experience and medical intuition when making a diagnosis, to the extent that clinical judgement can override formal diagnostic criteria in some circumstances. Psychological traditions from psychoanalysis through to person-centred and experiential therapies place great emphasis on clinical intuition, guiding therapists to 'trust' their feelings (i.e., empathic attunement) and intuitions about their patients (i.e., countertransference reactions). Although clinical intuition certainly plays an important role in the assessment and treatment process, it is also limited and error-prone. Several decades of research demonstrate that psychometric data-driven methods are superior to clinical judgement across a wide array of diagnostic and prognostic tasks (Ægisdóttir et al., 2006; Garb, 2005; Grove & Meehl, 1996; Grove et al., 2000). Diagnostic judgements are highly variable between different therapists, whereas structured diagnostic interviews and algorithms are highly consistent. Furthermore, it is notoriously difficult for therapists to predict their patients' treatment outcomes (Hannan et al., 2005), whereas data-driven and psychometric methods can be impressively accurate at predicting the future probability of deterioration (Finch et al., 2001) or symptomatic improvement (Bone et al., 2021). The evidence in this field is well-established by now, and the weight of evidence indicates that mental health professionals should use psychometric and data-driven methods to minimize errors of clinical judgement, particularly in relation to diagnosis and prognosis (i.e., assessing treatment response). As such, the omniscience fallacy is the product of a general tendency to rely on one's own intuition. Errors in detecting cases that tend to deteriorate are also explained by a general tendency for therapists to be optimistic about their effectiveness and their patient's likely outcomes. This optimistic attitude is of course necessary and important, as it enables therapists to retain and to instil a sense of hope in the likelihood of improvement, but it has the side effect of not being able to easily detect cases that are at high risk of deterioration. Over-optimism, negative attitudes to measurement and a general preference for relying on clinical judgement are well-known barriers to outcome monitoring (Jensen-Doss & Hawley, 2010).

The following solutions could be helpful to rectify such educational and attitudinal issues:

- Clinical supervisors should explore their supervisee's attitudes towards outcome measurement and monitoring and should encourage them to become familiar with this literature and the good practice guidelines outlined in this chapter.
- A useful exercise that therapists can carry out in order to assess and modify their beliefs and attitudes towards routine outcome monitoring is the following.
  - Make a prognostic assessment about every patient's likely outcome after treatment (reliable improvement, no reliable change, reliable deterioration, based on the reliable change index of the selected measure). This prognosis should ideally be made after having met the patient and assessed them (i.e., after two meetings). Keep a record of your prognostic assessment.
  - At the end of treatment, work out the observed outcome (reliable improvement, no reliable change, reliable deterioration) based on the reliable change index of the selected measure and make a record. Do this for a sufficient period of time to accumulate predicted and observed outcomes data for a number of cases (i.e., 10 or more).
  - Compare the absolute percentage of 'hits' and 'misses' between the expected and observed outcomes. Reflect on the extent to which clinical judgement accurately identifies those who improve, those who don't change, and those who deteriorate. This can be a useful task to carry out as part of clinical supervision, clinical training or team-based learning and development. A more extensive version of this exercise is proposed by Miller et al. (2020) as a starting point for learning from your outcomes and engaging in deliberate practice.

I sometimes have a tendency to think: 'I have been a psychologist for so many years, surely I can spot it when people are struggling with something.' But sometimes that turns out to be not quite the case. I had a patient who was on

the waiting list for therapy elsewhere and asked if I could do a bridging contact for 2–3 months. I took a very pragmatic approach, thinking I didn't need the ROM because it would only be a short treatment anyway. The patient was someone with whom it was difficult to make contact and who did not show much of herself in the therapy sessions. Just before she was transferring, she conducted a suicide attempt. I had completely missed it. If I had used ROM, I would have been able to see from the risk questions that suicidality was an issue. Fortunately, the attempt ended well, but I did think, 'Damn, I actually had the tools available to do this differently'.
— Anonymous cognitive behavioural therapist, the Netherlands

The ostrich syndrome

Even if therapists are versed in the literature on clinical judgement, ROM and feedback, it is easy to fall prey to the *ostrich syndrome*. The ostrich syndrome is a form of failure aversion, where people prefer not to be aware of problems in order to avoid feeling like a failure or accepting that things are not going as well as hoped. It is related to the psychoanalytic notion of *denial* (a defence mechanism) and the cognitive psychology concept of *selective abstraction*. Psychotherapists are particularly prone to this form of bias, as demonstrated by research showing that therapists are optimistically biased in their expectations about treatment progress and especially poor at predicting adverse treatment outcomes (Hannan et al., 2005). In practice, the ostrich syndrome takes the form of selective attention to information from outcome measures that indicates improvement, and selective dismissal or minimization of information that indicates no change or deterioration. A classic indicator of the ostrich syndrome is rationalizations of poor treatment response, such as:

- *'The measure is wrong, inaccurate, not measuring what really matters.'*
- *'The patient is not deteriorating. S/he is experiencing profound changes that are expected to be difficult and therefore show up as increased symptoms but are actually signs of improvement.'*
- *'Patients often get worse before they get better; improvements are expected to occur later on, in the longer term.'*
- *'Even though symptoms and functioning did not improve, the patient gained a lot from treatment in domains that were not measured, such as insight, personality change, self-acceptance, acceptance of their problems, etc.'*
- *'Even though symptoms or functioning did not improve, the patient reports being highly satisfied with treatment.'*

Rationalizations such as those illustrated above safeguard the therapist's sense of self-efficacy and perception of competence, which are important personal goals that support their well-being and confidence, but this comes at the expense of their patients' well-being and functioning. The exercise described in the above point (systematic comparison of predicted and observed outcomes) can be a useful way to correct this form of bias in order to make best use of routine outcome monitoring and feedback, which is known to be especially helpful to identify and work through cases with poor response to treatment.

> *One of the biggest challenges for me in using ROM and feedback is to truly want to receive feedback and to fight the temptation to correct the patient or to insist that I am 'right'. It is really humbling.*
> – Anonymous humanistic therapist, USA

Excessive agreeableness

While the ostrich syndrome is characterized by overly confident therapists who are motivated to attend to information that supports their sense of self-efficacy and to ignore and dismiss signals of treatment failure, sometimes therapists can have the opposite problem: a conscious awareness that therapy is not going well but a strong reluctance to deal with this in a timely way. Literature in the field of personality psychology indicates that people that are excessively *agreeable* (one of the *big five* personality traits) are highly accommodating in situations of intense emotional activation, and they tend to avoid confrontation and conflict at all costs (Perunovic & Holmes, 2008). Studies in the field of psychotherapy suggest that excessively agreeable therapists tend to have lower than average levels of patient-reported alliance ratings (Chapman et al., 2009) and poorer treatment outcomes (Delgadillo et al., 2020). Agreeableness is characterized by a prosocial, cooperative, considerate, likeable, trustful and empathic personality. Many of these facets of agreeableness are well-suited to the helping professions in general, and to psychotherapy in particular. However, excessive agreeableness is also characterized by *compliance* (an acquiescent and non-antagonistic orientation), which was found to be associated with poor treatment process and outcome measures in the studies cited above.

Literature in the field of psychotherapy indicates that the use of outcome measures and feedback is particularly important and effective when therapy is not on track. Thus, attending to these cases, discussing obstacles to improvement and finding a way forward are crucial to effective therapy. These tasks are not easy, and they can be emotionally challenging. It is easier to ignore problems, even if it is obvious that they are there. Excessive agreeableness can prevent therapists opening up a dialogue about problems in therapy, even when the problems are evident to the therapist. Potential solutions to this tendency to avoid difficult conversations can be to:

- Practise opening up discussions about poor treatment response through role-play exercises with a peer or clinical supervisor. Repeated practice should make it easier to desensitize to the emotional arousal that often accompanies these tasks.
- Record your therapy sessions and replay them in clinical supervision to obtain feedback from a clinical supervisor. This can help to identify situations where opportunities to address difficulties in-session were missed and to brainstorm ideas about how to intervene in a timely and sensitive way.

- Practise noticing your emotional, somatic and cognitive reactions to therapy situations where you notice yourself becoming overly compliant and avoiding difficult conversations with your patients. Train yourself to override these reactions and to intervene with a well-rehearsed dialogue that you can practise with your peers or supervisor in preparation for therapy sessions, with the goal of initiating and sustaining a conversation about problems in therapy. Examples of such dialogues are found in Chapter 8 of this book.

Supervisees often bring cases in which there is no improvement. There's trouble in compliance, the patient is complaining, worsening, or cancelling frequently. I often ask my supervisees: "Why don't you stop? Why go on with something that doesn't work?" And then they reply: "Well, the protocol should work for this patient, and I feel like I understand the patient and I would really like them to improve." "Sure, but if it does not work, it does not work. You work very hard on it. It gives you stress. It costs a lot of money. And the waiting list is still full." And when they discuss stopping, most patients actually respond that they agree, and were wondering for a while already if the therapy was still helpful. They appreciate you, the therapist, for bringing it up.
– Hidde Kuiper, CBT therapist and supervisor, the Netherlands

Inconsistency in the use of outcome measures

Other common problems that interfere with therapists' effective use of ROM and feedback are related to scheduling and discipline. Therapists can easily forget to prompt patients to complete outcome measures in a timely way, can forget to score and evaluate these measures, or to make time in-session to properly attend to routine outcome monitoring. These mistakes are much more common when therapists have busy schedules and little preparation time before starting their clinical working day or in between seeing patients. These small scheduling and memory lapses have a cumulative influence on the therapy process. If the therapist does not routinely attend to the measures, patients may not think they are important and may not feel motivated to complete them accurately. Furthermore, missed measurements also carry the risk of missed opportunities to identify and resolve obstacles to improvement, or to reinforce important positive changes that may have occurred relative to prior sessions. To a large extent, these practical lapses also have practical solutions such as:

- Asking patients to complete paper-and-pen questionnaires as soon as they arrive at the clinic reception area, where printed copies can be regularly kept or distributed by a receptionist.
- Automating the administration of outcome measures in a fixed schedule, using online surveys, mobile text or email-based questionnaires.
- Agreeing to spend the first five minutes of each session completing measures together, in the clinic room. Since this can take time away from other aspects of the therapy session agenda, this is only advisable if patients require help to complete questionnaires due to language comprehension or

literacy problems. This can also be appropriate with children and young people who may have a lower reading age or underdeveloped literacy skills.

- Keeping a visual aide-mémoire in your clinic room, such as a printed sheet that contains useful information about the interpretation rules (i.e., scoring procedures, cut-off scores, reliable change index) for outcome measures, in a highly visible place.

> *Incorporate it into your own routine. I put in my intake form in big letters that I ask people if they want to fill out the ROM. It's also in my consent form. Then the chances increase incrementally that you will do it.*
> – Erik van der Put, private practitioner and CBT therapist, the Netherlands

Patient-related difficulties

Forgetting to complete measures

A common problem, especially during the earliest sessions of therapy, is that the patient may forget to complete measures before their therapy appointment. This is understandable, since it is a new and unfamiliar task. Like any other new behavioural repertoire, outcome measurement needs to be reinforced in order to become learned, and we can employ basic principles of learning theory and contingency management to achieve this. Some strategies to support and reinforce the adoption of outcome measurement are the following:

- *Priming*: Simple strategies such as setting a weekly reminder using a phone, text messages or email reminders can be easily automated using modern technology. Ideally, reminders that prime the patient to complete measures before the start of their session should be scheduled in a consistent manner, so as to support their integration into the patient's therapy and weekly routine.
- *Cue retrieval*: It can be useful to have copies of questionnaires or results visible to the patient during the therapy session (i.e. paper-based questionnaires/printed results visibly laid out on a table, or a graphical display of outcome measures or feedback systems on a computer screen). Through associative learning, the patient would integrate the measurement aspects of treatment within their wider network of associations and cues about therapy (i.e. 'therapy involves the therapist, the therapy consulting room, the measures, the computer, etc.'). If this associative learning takes place, it would make it easier for the patient to think about completing the measures when they start to think about attending their next therapy appointment.
- *Positive reinforcement*: Crucial to the success of the above strategies is the need to positively reinforce the completion of outcome measures. This is especially important during the earliest appointments, and can be accomplished by: (1) thanking the patient for remembering to complete the measures;

(2) spending time to review, interpret and integrate results from measures into the therapy session; (3) referring to the measures during the therapy session, whenever specific symptoms/goals come up in conversation, so as to draw attention to the connection between the patient's dialogue/concerns/goals and the information captured in the measures (this enhances the patient's perception of the face validity and relevance of the measure to their concerns).

- *Negative reinforcement*: If none of the above strategies work, and the patient continues to forget completing measures, negative reinforcement can be used carefully. The goal of this approach is to introduce a mild form of 'penalty' whenever the patient forgets to complete the measure, and which the patient would seek to avoid in the future by completing the measure in a timely way. A mild 'penalty', for example, would be for the therapist to politely ask the patient to quietly complete the measure in session, during the first few minutes before making a start with the session (the time taken up by completing a measure within the session could be perceived as a mild 'penalty'). However, we emphasize that the use of negative reinforcement is not advisable as a first choice of strategy, since it could make the process of outcome measurement aversive for some patients (especially if they have difficulties with reading, writing, language barriers, etc.) and can be perceived as taking away the autonomy of the patient on completing a measure or not. It is important to also remember that, according to learning theory, 'negative reinforcement' is not the same as 'punishment'. Negative reinforcement is a process where an action is learned and repeated in order to avoid some kind of hassle or undesirable consequence. Once the action has been learned and established as part of the therapy routine, the therapist should resort to positive reinforcement methods thereafter, as outlined above.

Literacy problems

As alluded to in the previous point, some patients may have difficulties related to literacy, comprehension and language barriers, or may struggle to read printed or electronic materials for other reasons (e.g., eye-sight problems). In these circumstances, the following strategies can help to increase the accessibility and acceptability of routine outcome monitoring:

- Ask the patient if specific adjustments can make questionnaires more accessible, such as printing in a specific background colour, using a specific font size, using audio-recorded questions, etc.
- Obtain translated measures in the person's primary language
- Enlist the help of a trusted family member or friend who can support the person to complete measures prior to attending sessions
- Select and use measures with a minimal number of items (i.e., ultra-brief validated versions of lengthier questionnaires)
- Completing the measures in the form of an interview during the first part of each therapy session, completed by the therapist.

Of course, the option in the last bullet point can be time-consuming. Therefore, other options listed above should be explored first, and this can be seen as a last resort which needs to be conducted in a sensitive and conversational way that fully integrates the process of measurement with the therapy dialogue and session, so that it is experienced as part of the therapy itself rather than a burdensome task that gets in the way of starting the therapy session.

Resistance

It is widely documented in the psychotherapy literature that sometimes we encounter patients who are reluctant to engage in therapy tasks that may be theoretically and/or empirically advisable to be a part of their treatment plan. In what concerns outcome monitoring, this 'resistance' can take the form of neglecting (i.e., 'I didn't have time to do it; I couldn't be bothered to do it') or outrightly refusing to complete outcome measures. If this occurs, an insistence from the part of the therapist to complete measures could lead to an alliance rupture. Thus, the nature of the resistance should be sensitively explored, understood and addressed. Sometimes this 'resistance' could be explained by the following:

• The patient does not fully understand why they are being asked to complete the measure repeatedly. This would require revisiting the rationale for routine outcome monitoring, using metaphors to explain its purpose, as described earlier in this chapter.

• The patient does not consider this to be important for their therapy. Further to restating the rationale for outcome monitoring, a clear explanation that this form of feedback can actually help to improve the patient's health and problems could serve to emphasize and reinforce their commitment to this process.

• The patient's main problems and concerns are not reflected in the outcome measure. This would require considering and selecting another measure that has greater face validity for the patient.

• The patient feels anxious about what the results might reveal, or anxious about the consequences of endorsing certain items (i.e., suicidal ideas, self-harm, anger, etc.). This requires having a dialogue about how these symptoms are quite common, that they can improve, and that being able to talk about them and track them is an essential part of the treatment process. In particular, it is crucial that the therapist addresses this topic by showing compassion and empathy towards the patient, validating their anxiety/fears, and assuring them that they are doing the right thing by divulging this information and bringing it to therapy.

• The patient believes that they are a failure, and will fail at therapy, and the measures will show this failure. As described above, a sensitive and compassionate stance towards validating the patient's concerns is required to deal with this issue. Furthermore, some psychoeducation could also be helpful to enable the patient to learn that these symptoms and problems actually fluctuate over time in most cases, they tend to improve during therapy, and can improve considerably if feedback is used in order to support and inform the treatment plan. The therapist could use anonymized outcome monitoring charts from previous cases to illustrate this point.

A more complicated form of resistance is documented in Larry Beutler's research on the concept of 'reactance'. According to Beutler et al. (2018), reactance is an interpersonal style whereby the person has a lack of an inclination to change and is strongly invested in opposing those who seek to change them. In theory, the primary motivation for this oppositional stance is to preserve one's sense of mastery and independence. Clinical trials show that highly reactant patients respond less favourably to highly directive interventions, whereas they respond better to less directive approaches which enable them to preserve their sense of agency. This requires a subtle negotiation with patients, whereby the goal of routine outcome monitoring is achieved, but in such a way that preserves the patient's sense of agency and which is carried out based on their preferences and 'on their terms'. Some strategies to achieve this are listed below:

- Come up with a set of potential measures to choose from. Ask the patient to choose the one they prefer and which makes most sense to them.
- Offer a set of choices around the timing (day/time) and format (paper, text message, online) for routine outcome monitoring. Make those choices more diverse than you would usually offer other patients; the goal is to create an atmosphere where the patient gets the impression that they are in control and that they are refusing several unfit choices and going with the one that they prefer.
- Avoid using excessive praise or positive reinforcement (i.e., 'thank you for taking time to complete the measure today'), which could be perceived as patronizing by reactant patients. It is better to deal with the outcome monitoring and interpretation in a business-like way, signalling to the patient that they are in charge of the process and the therapist is providing them with a service that adjusts to their preferences.
- Always be consistent in following through a structured routine of gathering, attending to, interpreting and discussing the results of outcome measures. Deviations from this routine could signal to a reactant patient that the therapist is in charge of when to attend to this information or when to ignore it and the patient may feel suspicious or uncomfortable about this perceived imbalance of control.

We had a patient in our clinic who had complained to their therapist that they were only caring about the numbers on the questionnaire and not about him. So, the therapist brought it up in supervision and said: "Well, I think I need to stop using the ROM and feedback, as the patient does not like it." And the thing is, in those cases, the response of the patient is not really about the assessment, but rather it is an indication that the patient felt neglected – that he wanted to be cared for. And if you address that, the ROM itself will no longer be a problem.

*– Wolfgang Lutz, feedback researcher and
CBT therapist, Germany*

Mindless or stereotyped responding

Sometimes, patients complete questionnaires as fast as possible, without paying too much attention to the items, or without thinking about or following the specific instructions for that measure. Sometimes patients provide the same responses every single week, as if they had memorized their initial responses and follow the same blueprint thereafter in a stereotyped way. Other times patients show extreme response styles, where they choose either the highest or the lowest response option consistently, in a mechanical way. This sort of 'mindless responding' obviously leads to inaccuracies in the measurement of their health indicators. Some strategies to deal with this are as follows:

- Check if the patient fully understands the instructions and the meaning of each item in the questionnaire. Mindless responding can sometimes reveal literacy or comprehension problems.
- Check if the patient feels anxious when they complete the measure. Mindless responding can sometimes reveal anxious expectations or failure aversion, as described in the previous point.
- Train the patient to 'slow down' using this sequence: (1) read the instructions out loud, (2) form an image of yourself in your own mind related to the questionnaire item and the time-frame indicated by the instructions; (3) answer the first item; (4) form an image of yourself in your own mind related to the next questionnaire item and the timeframe indicated by the instructions; (5) complete the next item; (6) repeat the prior steps until you finish all items. This exercise is usually only necessary to carry out once or twice, until the patient has learned to grasp the meaning of the items, the specific timeframe for evaluation and the sequence of items. Thereafter, the process of self-monitoring tends to become less stereotyped.

Motivated responding

Sometimes patients fully understand the instructions, the meaning of the questionnaire items and the rationale for outcome monitoring and feedback, but they still provide stereotyped responses that indicate extreme states (i.e., extremely mild or extremely severe symptoms) or a state that does not seem to correspond with the patient's demeanour and self-reported functioning (i.e., measuring high levels of PTSD, but not reporting any recent intrusive memories, related distress or avoidance of triggers). Sometimes this can be explained by 'motivated responding', which is when a patient is motivated to provide an inaccurate measure because it either leads to some form of gain or prevents some form of loss. Some examples of such motives are listed below.

- *Social desirability bias*: The patient is highly motivated to please the therapist and to provide answers that they perceive to be the type of answers that the therapist wants to see, or that will make the therapist look good (in a managed health system). In this case, the patient may actually not be well, but they may respond in such a way that downplays their distress. As such, recognizing this and addressing this as a particular interpersonal process would be an important task for the therapist.

- *Secondary gains*: The patient is unwell, and they are not motivated to change, because being and remaining unwell is reinforced by interpersonal (i.e., sickness elicits compassion, care, company), financial (i.e., disability or sickness payment), or other gains (i.e., being sick legitimizes their position in a social or peer group and provides a sense of identity and value). Similarly, recognizing this and addressing this as a particular interpersonal process would be an important task for the therapist, and could be a good target for a decisional balance exercise and motivational interviewing techniques.

- *Gaming*: The patient is not unwell (i.e., they do not meet criteria for a mental health problem), but they respond to questionnaires as if they were unwell, because this may render some of the gains listed above. Again, recognizing this and addressing this as a particular interpersonal process would be an important task for the therapist, and could be addressed using motivational interviewing techniques in order to come to a decision about whether or not therapy is appropriate.

- *Separation anxiety and dependency*: The patient provides consistently elevated measures of distress or dysfunction, related to anxiety about finishing therapy, feeling highly dependent or attached to the therapist, or other concerns related to themes of abandonment or loss. Sometimes this form of separation anxiety becomes evident at later stages of therapy, after some improvements have been made and when the therapy process moves into the phase of planning the end of treatment in short-term or time-limited interventions. Often this is explicit in a patient's communications to the therapist, for example if they state they fear getting worse or not being able to cope without therapy. Sometimes this separation anxiety can manifest in signals of neediness or dependence, for example if the patient demands longer sessions, or more frequent sessions than previously agreed, or the patient makes unplanned contacts requesting advice or support (i.e., emails, phone calls, telephone messages). This can in turn evoke extreme emotional reactions in the therapist, either as enmeshment (i.e., feeling a need to rescue the patient) or disengagement (i.e., feeling burdened and needing some distance). As described above, recognizing this interpersonal process would be an important task for the therapist and could be discussed explicitly in order to promote insight about how such an interpersonal process may be related to the patient's interpersonal history, needs and current problems.

I use ROM and feedback as an intervention as well as evaluation of the progress of the therapy. I had a patient who was in a very bad condition at the start of treatment. He improved due to medication and therapy, and he loved the therapy more and more. So, he gave me the impression that he wanted to stay in therapy. He came up with all kinds of new issues that he wanted to discuss and he really enjoyed it. So, we did the ROM and I noticed that there was progress in the beginning and then it stabilized. So, I discussed this with my patient

and I said: "I'm worried, because there is no more progress." And he said: "No, there still is progress!". And I said: "Well, if there is no more progress, we should discuss ending the therapy." He responded with "No, I don't want to end the therapy." So, it was right on the button. I said: "If there is no progress observable in the ROM scores, then I have to end the therapy." The next time he completed the ROM, his scores had improved incredibly and was well under the cutoff for caseness. So, I said to him: "Wow, what a finish! So now we can end the therapy." He did not look very happy, but he had to acknowledge that it was the end. So, for me, it really is an intervention.
– Hidde Kuiper, CBT therapist, the Netherlands

An important common theme across the examples above is that ROM and feedback are valuable tools for communication. If patients fail to complete measures, this tells us something about the patient's adherence to the therapy process. If patients complete measures in a way that seems inaccurate or discrepant with our observations and other data sources, this reveals the presence of misunderstandings or motivated responding. Completing or refusing to complete measures is an act of communication, and what matters is to work with the patient to understand what is being communicated. In the absence of the above types of difficulties, when patients complete measures accurately and consistently, the scores serve as a useful index of treatment progress or deterioration. As such, a central question that every therapist that is committed to the use of routine outcome monitoring should always have in mind is: what is the patient communicating?

Conclusions

Although the implementation of ROM and feedback seems like something that could be relatively straightforward, in practice it is not an easy task. Apart from barriers and enablers at the organizational level, which have been discussed in Chapter 3, therapists and patients may also have cognitions and attitudes that may help or hinder the implementation of ROM and feedback. In Chapter 3, we discussed how a creating a culture of feedback is an important part of successful long-term implementation. Once such a culture has been established, many of the issues presenting in this chapter will fall away, as therapists and patients will get used to working with ROM and feedback as an integral part of therapy. Therapists will automatically use the output and ask for it when it is not available, and because they get better at explaining it, patients will also be more convinced that it is a useful part of therapy.

Key points in this chapter

- Realize that there is no such thing as the perfect outcome measure, but rather choose the one that best fits your practice.

- Working with ROM and feedback can trigger avoidance tendencies and/or defence mechanisms in therapists as well as patients.
- Response tendencies in patients may reduce the validity of the ROM measurements and should be addressed with the patient if they come up in the discussion of the feedback. In discussing them, try to keep in mind what the patient is trying to communicate through their responses.

5 Introducing routine outcome monitoring to patients

In this chapter

Previous chapters focused on the science behind routine outcome monitoring (ROM) and provided information on how to select, implement and interpret outcome measures in routine clinical practice. This chapter provides a practical guide on how to introduce outcome measures to patients, with a particular focus on early sessions of therapy because establishing ROM as an integral part of practice at the beginning is most likely to yield the maximum benefit. Examples are provided on how to explain the rationale for outcome monitoring in a way that promotes patients' adherence to the process.

Always introduce feedback at the start of therapy

Routine outcome monitoring is an integral part of effective and evidence-based therapy. As such, it is important to introduce it and orient patients to this practice at the earliest stages of therapy. There are four important reasons to introduce this at the initial therapy session with every new patient.

First, reliable outcome monitoring requires a pre-treatment measure to interpret the patient's response over time with reference to this baseline. The baseline measure captures critical information about the patient's level of distress preceding the formal start of treatment, since most psychometric questionnaires used in clinical practice require the respondent to assess their symptoms retrospectively, for example in the preceding weeks or month. This pre-treatment measure usually conveys information about the peak level of distress that we might expect to observe during treatment, since significant deterioration compared with this baseline measure over the course of treatment is uncommon (e.g., 10 per cent or fewer patients) and would be an important signal that treatment is not working well. Without a baseline measure, the therapist does not have a clear sense about the peak level of distress, and is less able to accurately judge if an intensification of distress is indeed a signal of poor response to treatment or simply a natural fluctuation that is in accordance with typical treatment response.

Second, if outcome monitoring is introduced sometime after the start of therapy, valuable information about early response is lost. As discussed in Chapter 4, early response is one of the most well-established prognostic indicators and changes that occur in the early stages of treatment account for a large proportion of the overall change that early responders attain throughout treatment. Assessing if reliable improvement has occurred or not during the first four sessions of treatment provides valuable information about the patient's treatment response. If outcome monitoring is introduced late, say at sessions three or four, the therapist may be unaware of symptomatic changes that occurred after the first couple of sessions, and which may possibly account for a significant percentage of the overall change for that patient. In such circumstances, where a patient experiences considerable early change in the first few sessions, the data from the remaining trajectory of outcome monitoring may give the appearance of limited change.

Third, as discussed in previous chapters, most computerized feedback systems generate interpretation rules such as expected treatment response (ETR) curves or early response signals that are based on the pre-treatment baseline measure. Without capturing a pre-treatment baseline, it is not possible to use some of the most widely available computerized feedback systems.

Fourth, the effective use of ROM and feedback involves having discussions with patients about their progress in therapy. Sometimes, as discussed in Chapter 7, this involves discussing situations when treatment may not be working well. Raising this discussion later on in therapy can be alarming to some patients if it seems unexpected. It is therefore crucial to appropriately orient patients to the purpose, structure and use of ROM and feedback as part of therapy. If patients understand that treatment progress will be regularly monitored, assessed and openly discussed with them, potentially difficult conversations become expected and less alarming.

In summary, it is essential to gather a pre-treatment baseline measure to effectively integrate ROM and feedback into clinical practice and to use available computerized feedback systems. In the following sections, we provide practical guidelines on how to introduce patients to ROM and feedback in the earliest sessions of therapy.

Explaining the rationale for routine outcome monitoring

It is important to provide a clear rationale for ROM and feedback, to enable the patient to ask questions, and to discuss and resolve any concerns that they may have. Ideally, this should be accomplished as part of the initial session to collaboratively agree how therapy will work and what it will involve in the subsequent sessions. However, exactly when and how this is done in the first session is something for each therapist to decide on the basis of their own therapeutic approach but also, importantly, the present state of the individual patient. As a general principle, the patient's responses to outcome measures

Box 5.1 Discussing the rationale for ROM and feedback

T: An important part of treatment involves keeping track of your difficulties over time, so that we can get a sense of how treatment is working and if it is helping you to feel better or not. We use some questionnaires to do this. Were you able to complete the questionnaire you received before this appointment?

P: Ah yes, here it is.

T: Great, thank you. Before we have a look at it together, maybe I can explain why you were asked to complete this.

P: OK.

T: Health care providers commonly use measures to assess health problems. For example, a doctor might take your temperature using a thermometer if you have a fever. The doctor might prescribe some form of treatment to help with this. If the treatment works, we would expect that the fever calms down, and one easy way to check this is to take another measure of your temperature and to compare it to the initial measure. Does that make sense to you?

P: Um… yes, I see what you mean.

T: This questionnaire is like a sort of thermometer for mental health problems.

P: Right, I see…

T: Thermometers and questionnaires are certainly not perfect. But the results are still quite useful, because they give us a general sense of the intensity of the underlying problem. Like temperature, mental health problems usually fluctuate in intensity and change over time.

P: Yes, my problems seem to go up and down. Some days are worse than others.

T: Exactly. We can use this questionnaire to keep track of changes in your level of distress during the course of therapy and to adjust the treatment to make sure it works as well as possible for you. Would you be willing to complete this before the start of every session? Is that OK with you?

P: OK, sure.

T: Great, thank you. Now let's have a look at the questionnaire together and I can explain how to interpret it…

should be integrated into the session material, as part of the therapy dialogue. An example of a dialogue aiming to explain the rationale is illustrated in the vignette in Box 5.1.

The example in Box 5.1 illustrates good practice principles in routine outcome monitoring:

- *Explain the purpose*: it helps to track progress.
- *Personalise it*: it matters to you, because it is about your difficulties and your well-being.
- *Use familiar concepts to make it seem familiar straight away*: choose one or more metaphors that convey the notions of measurement and change.

- *Use scaffolding*: once a familiar concept has been discussed, link this familiar concept to the concept of routine outcome monitoring.
- *Check understanding and clarify*: ask questions to obtain feedback from the patient, to ensure that they understand the rationale and to open up an opportunity to clarify any questions.
- *Set expectations*: prepare the patient to be ready to complete measures regularly, underlining the purpose of doing this.
- *Interpret and share information*: explain how you interpret the measure and how it is informative for the treatment plan.

Analogies, metaphors and scaffolding

Using familiar concepts and scaffolding are two of the most important principles outlined above, since they will enable the patient to easily understand the purpose of completing measures and, therefore, to build motivation and commitment to this aspect of treatment. Analogies (drawing a parallel between two concepts) and metaphors (using symbolism and figurative language) can be useful in this regard, but this doesn't always 'work' if it is not attuned to the patient's concerns and viewpoint. For an analogy or a metaphor to be effective, it must be intuitive and familiar to the patient and it should carry implicit meaning about the concepts of measurement and change.

With the wider implementation of psychological therapies to diverse settings, countries and populations, the field has become increasingly aware of and responsive to issues related to diversity and multicultural sensitivity. For example, research indicates that cultural adaptations to psychological therapy can help to make therapy more effective for patients from racial and ethnic minorities (e.g., Hall et al., 2016). In particular, explaining concepts of mental health problems and related treatment strategies using language and metaphors that are sensitive to the patient's cultural context and worldview can support the development of a working alliance and foster engagement with the treatment (Benish et al., 2011).

An effective metaphor promotes new learning using the principle of *scaffolding*, which refers to building new knowledge on top of available knowledge. The thermometer analogy illustrated in Box 5.1 achieves this by appealing to widely familiar concepts: a thermometer is a measurement tool, it measures temperature, there are different levels of temperature, high temperature usually signifies an undesirable state, temperature fluctuates, it is common to measure temperature repeatedly if one has a fever, health care providers use thermometers, etc. This analogy is packed full of implicit concepts and knowledge for many ordinary people who are familiar with health care practices. Although this is an analogy that makes sense to many people, therapists can use a wide range of other concepts to achieve the same goal. Examples of other concepts are provided below, mainly to illustrate that therapists can and should be creative and flexible in the way in which they introduce the rationale for

ROM and feedback. These examples are selected to be relevant to a wide range of problems commonly encountered in clinical practice.

- *Depression*: 'Sometimes depression can feel like an enormous weight that holds people down and prevents them from living the life they want to live. This questionnaire is like a scale that measures how heavy your depression has been recently. That way, we can keep track of it over time, to get a sense of whether therapy is helping to ease the load of depression and to make it feel less heavy.'
- *Intrusive memories, thoughts or voices*: 'Sometimes mental health problems can be like an overwhelming noise in your mind, with negative or disturbing thoughts that get really loud. We use this questionnaire to get a sense of how loud and overwhelming the mental distress is. That way, we can keep track of this over time, to get a sense of whether therapy is helping to regulate the volume or not. We wouldn't expect the noise to be eliminated altogether, but we can certainly try to regulate it and reduce the volume to a tolerable level'.
- *Disturbing or overwhelming emotions*: 'Mental health problems can often feel like you're constantly caught up in a storm, and this can feel scary and unsafe. One way to see if therapy is helping with this is to keep track of the storm. We can use a questionnaire to do this. It's like a barometer of your internal weather. Like the external weather, mental distress comes and goes, and it changes with the seasons. We want to get to that point, where the storm calms down and the weather seems more variable rather than always unsafe.'
- *Compulsive or addictive behaviours*: 'Sometimes people experience this problem as if their brain is split into two parts. One compulsive side of your brain is pushing you to do this, while the adaptive side of your brain knows that this causes you problems and suffering. At the moment it must feel like the compulsive side is stronger, but therapy can help to train the adaptive side to the point where it becomes stronger than the compulsive side. The tricky thing is that we can't directly see these sides of your brain, but we can measure their influence on your behaviour using a questionnaire. It's like a strength meter for the compulsive side of your brain.'

As illustrated in the above examples, effective analogies and metaphors serve as an explanatory device, not only to convey the principles of measurement during therapy, but also to promote insight into the natural progression of a mental health problem, its expected fluctuations and realistic expectations about the outcomes of treatment. In this way, routine outcome monitoring is as much part of the treatment itself (i.e., this dialogue promotes insight and influences positive expectancies) as it is a process of feedback and evaluation. As such, the choice of metaphor has to be adjusted to each individual patient's circumstances and particularities of their presenting problems.

Metaphors for children or adults with limited literacy skills, for example, should be straightforward and uncomplicated. The figures of speech represented in the metaphor (e.g., scales to measure weight, a ruler to measure the depth of a hole) should correspond to figures of speech in common parlance (e.g., I'm weighed down by depression, I'm down in the dumps) or which align to the person's cultural or religious worldview if relevant. More concrete language (e.g., 'this questionnaire gives us a score for how unwell you feel, where a high score is really difficult and a low score is OK') should be used in situations where the patient may think in a more concrete way and may find metaphors overly abstract or confusing. Similarly, in the context of therapy for children, it is common to collect information and feedback from multiple perspectives (i.e., the child, a parent, a teacher), and therefore an adjustment of the use of language and metaphors for each perspective is crucial to effective communication and outcome measurement. Overall, flexibility and personalization are key to the success of an effective metaphor and rationale.

Interpreting routine outcome measures

After discussing the rationale for routine outcome monitoring, it is important to take some time to explain how the relevant questionnaire is interpreted and how it might inform the treatment process. This is usually accomplished at the first or second therapy session, depending on time availability. In particular, if this is done at the first therapy session, it is important to accomplish it in a small amount of time, because patients are usually eager to explain their difficulties and hear about what therapy involves, rather than to spend too much time on technical aspects of outcome measurement. This explanation generally involves answering the three following questions as part of a dialogue with the patient:

* How are the questionnaire results worked out?
* How are they interpreted in a clinical way?
* How can this information be helpful for the patient?

The first point involves explaining the scoring or classification rules for the relevant questionnaire. The second point involves explaining the clinical norms used to interpret a specific score and changes in this score over time. The third point underlines key issues that are particularly relevant to the patient and which might become targets for treatment or salient indicators for routine outcome monitoring. Box 5.2 provides an example illustrating all of these points based on the PHQ-9 depression questionnaire (Kroenke, Spitzer & Williams, 2001).

Explaining the interpretation of questionnaires is an important way to enable a transparent and collaborative process of outcome monitoring. It demystifies the outcome monitoring process and offers opportunities to gain insight into the specific problem domains that are most salient at a particular point in time. The attention to detail and interest that the therapist demonstrates as part of this dialogue implicitly reinforces the patient's commitment to the process: this process matters, it is personalized, interesting, purposeful and its ultimate goal is to illuminate the path towards improvement.

The same attention to detail and careful interpretation should be a hallmark of every subsequent therapy session. In this way, the patient's commitment to

---

Box 5.2 Explaining the interpretation of an outcome measure

T: Let's see. Based on your responses to this questionnaire, I have worked out a total score, which measures the intensity of your depression over the last two weeks. This score can range between 0 and 27. The higher the score, the more severe the problem. It's like a thermometer reading, but for low mood.

P: OK, I get it. So, what's my score?

T: Your score is fairly high, at 18, which means that you're having these symptoms quite regularly and it's become pretty difficult for you.

P: Yes, I'm finding it hard to deal with it most days.

T: Right, it's a heavy load that's holding you down most days... When people have scores above 20, we consider that severe depression, which usually stops people from being able to do most things in the usual way. Your score is close to 20, which shows that things are tough at the moment. I can also see that disrupted sleep, low energy and trouble concentrating are especially difficult.

P: Yes, it feels really tough. I can hardly focus because I'm exhausted due to insomnia.

T: Therapy can help with these problems. As we make progress with treatment, usually we expect to see these scores go down over time. A score below 10 usually indicates that the symptoms have reduced to a minimal and more manageable level...

---

and interest in the outcome monitoring process becomes reinforced and established as part of the expected role of the patient. In later sessions, it is advisable that the therapist reviews outcome measures with the patient as a standard part of the therapy session, ideally towards the beginning of each session. This ensures the continuous reinforcement of outcome monitoring as a shared task but also ensures that potential problems (i.e., symptomatic deterioration) can be prioritized and dealt with as part of the session, allowing sufficient time to deal with difficulties. Chapter 8 provides detailed guidelines on how to respond if patients' treatment response is not on track.

In many cases, subsequent measures are indicative of an expected treatment response or improvement, in which case the therapist can offer this interpretation, check the patient's perspective about this interpretation, and move on with the usual tasks and agenda for the therapy session. For instance, by saying, 'This week's scores are quite similar to last week, which might indicate that things haven't changed much with your mental health. Does that fit with your experience?' In this latter scenario, routine outcome monitoring tasks (reviewing, interpreting, and discussing the measures) do not usually take any more than a few minutes at the start of the therapy session. However, in the scenario where outcome measures indicate a statistically reliable improvement, this can be a highly valuable opportunity to use progress feedback to gain insights about key processes of change or contextual factors that might support improvements in the patient's mental health. Attending to specific items within the questionnaire – for instance noticing which ones changed more substantially than others since the last measurement – can promote insights into key problems and processes than enable change. For instance, the therapist could attend to this by saying, 'This week's scores seem considerably better than last week; I wonder if we can try to understand what might be explaining this positive change? Let's have a look at the pattern of these symptoms and compare them to last session. What are your thoughts about it?' In this way, the tasks of reviewing, interpreting, and learning from routine outcome measures become an integral part of the therapy and enable the therapist to be highly responsive to situations where the patient's mental health is improving, stagnating or deteriorating.

Conclusions

The clinical utility of routine outcome monitoring is largely dependent on complete, accurate and regularly available measures. In order to establish such a set of conditions, it is crucial to introduce outcome measures to patients in a way that will maximize their commitment to this process. Introducing outcome monitoring is not a simple task. It requires the therapist to have a good technical understanding of how to interpret measures clinically and an ability to explain this in a way that is attuned to each patient's life circumstances (i.e., age, mastery of language, cultural norms, etc.) and clinical presentation (i.e., symptoms, problems). If therapists introduce measurement early enough and in a way that supports adherence to the process, ROM and feedback becomes an integral part of each therapy session, without a need to be overly time consuming or burdensome. Most importantly, this enables therapists and patients to have a shared mechanism to discover what helps and hinders their treatment progress over the course of therapy.

Key points in this chapter

- Introduce the rationale for routine outcome monitoring at the earliest opportunity; ideally at the initial appointment.
- Use metaphors to explain the rationale for routine outcome monitoring.
- Patients should be guided on how to interpret measures, so that their interpretation can become a shared and collaborative task throughout treatment.
- Therapists should consistently attend to measures at regular intervals during therapy, so as to acknowledge, validate and reinforce the patient's commitment to this process.
- Overall, once a process of routine outcome monitoring becomes established, it can serve as a mechanism to learn about the factors that worsen, maintain or alleviate mental health problems.

6 Interpreting scores and patterns in measurements

As soon as you have collected your data, before you compute any statistics, look at your data.

(Wilkinson & Task Force on Statistical Inference, 1999, p. 597, emphasis in original)

In this chapter

In this chapter, we consider what data from ROM can tell you about a patient's psychological state and their progress in therapy. However, we start by discussing ROM at the initial session and how you can make best use of the information at this early stage. Subsequently, high frequency measurement data provide information that yield patterns that are signals regarding a patient's response and progress over time in therapy, and, accordingly, we focus on the various shapes of change that repeated sessional data display. In this chapter, we will focus on positive shapes of change and in Chapter 7 we will discuss shapes of change that demonstrate a lack of progress.

Interpreting ROM data from the initial session

While our major focus is on the use of *repeated* sessional data and its role in progress feedback, data completed at the *initial* session presents a slightly different situation in that there is no previous sessional data with which to make comparisons, although there may be data from an earlier assessment or screening. As such, it may appear that there is not much information to be gained by considering the data at this stage. However, similar to the process of therapy itself, the initial session has a central focus on engagement and it is important to use this opportunity to develop a culture or climate whereby ROM is seen and accepted by patients as integral to the therapeutic process.

Scanning the items

Each therapist will have their own approach as to how much they integrate the content of the measure into informing their in-session therapeutic work. One approach is to scan by eye the item scores and note, with the patient, those items that are marked as absent or low, or as high on distress (if a questionnaire measures functioning, high scores often refer to better functioning, which reverses the interpretation). For example: 'I notice that your scores on items x, y, and z are zero, meaning they have not been an issue for you this week. Is that right?' A key point here is that it is important to focus on positive outcomes as one key message to feed back to a patient is that there are aspects of life that are positive and that these are recognized in the therapy. Another approach is to draw attention to items, or selected items if there are many, where the patient is scoring high: 'I see that you have marked the maximum score for items x, y, and z. Would it be useful to use these as a starting point for our session today?' Of course, a therapist may have thought before the session about what the focus might be but, obviously, at the initial session there is no agenda set from the previous session. Accordingly, there is more freedom than usual, perhaps, for the therapist to utilize the information from the outcome measures.

There is also a further possible response that therapists might find useful, and that focuses on the phenomenon of missing data. When patients take part in a clinical trial and miss out on an item, this is invariably viewed as an error (e.g., data point missing at random). However, the value of missing data in clinical practice lies in what it is potentially saying about the patient. It might be that the patient is uncertain or unable to make a response; or it might be something specific that the patient has in mind when thinking about the item, that it conjures up a myriad of feelings that they want to turn away from. The take-home message here is that absence of data provides clinical information and should not immediately be viewed as error. Of course, if the data completion method is via an electronic device, it is likely that a patient will not be able to proceed to the next item or question without completing the current page. Hence, at one level, missing data does not occur. However, if one is minded that there is a component of choice when a patient completes an item, then a procedure that forces a person into providing a response may not be viewed so positively. So, while digital methods that ensure completion have some advantages, they can also mask subtle clinical issues that may be apparent when the patient has a choice regarding item completion. Interestingly, going the other way, in the future, it is possible that the increasing use of digital methods of data collection may provide information to the therapist on the time taken by the patient to complete each item, which might, in the future, be useful clinical information as to items that generated greater thought processing by the patient.

Overall, familiarity with the measure by the therapist is crucial as, with time and experience, a therapist will begin to develop the ability to recognize differing profiles of responses by eye-balling the completed measure. But a key point here is that the therapist must know the measure thoroughly, to maximize its yield but also to convey confidence in the measure to the patient.

Interpreting initial severity and symptom profile

While there may not be information on the change process at the initial session, one task that can be achieved at the initial session is get an idea of the severity of a patient's problems. For most measures used in ROM and feedback, there are normative scores available that help interpret the initial score by comparison to other patients (also discussed in Chapter 2). Hi-tech feedback systems will typically provide some sort of interpretation of the score already, but even in no-tech and lo-tech solutions, it is easy to keep a normative table from the measure's administration manual at hand, or copy it into the spreadsheet you use to monitor progress. Some manuals offer normative tables with percentile scores and you can compare your patient's score to them. For example, a score of 85 on a fictional outcome measure is located at the 90th percentile for outpatients. Other manuals offer classifications of severity; for example, a score between 21 and 30 is considered to be a moderate depression on the Beck Depression Inventory (Second Edition) (BDI-II; Beck et al., 1996).

Some outcome measures have multiple scales, which typically makes it worth looking at the pattern of the scales, identifying which ones are high, and which ones are low or moderate. In some cases, a general elevated pattern is visible, in which (almost) all subscales have relatively high scores, whereas in other cases there are some scales that are elevated, but others on which the patient does not have issues or is functioning well. You can have a conversation with the patient on what you notice as a therapist and whether the patient recognizes these patterns or not (see concrete examples in Chapters 4 and 5).

Furthermore, observing the pattern of item responses across a questionnaire can offer clinically useful information for discussion with the patient at the initial stage of therapy. For example, some specific problems may be more severe than others, and these could provide clues about the primary targets or issues to work on. For example, when treating a patient with social anxiety, a measure such as the Social Phobia Inventory (SPIN; Connor et al., 2000) could help the therapist to identify which specific types of situations are more relevant to a particular patient (e.g., public speaking, fear of blushing, fear of authority, etc.). Subsequent meetings at the later stages of therapy could enable both the therapist and patient to assess changes across these specific situations and to identify problems that have not yet improved and that could be specifically targeted. This attention to detail and focus on measures as a device to inform clinical discussions with the patient exemplifies how measures can be usefully integrated into the therapy process.

Components of meaningful (statistical) change

At the outset, it is worth stating that this text is very much focused on therapists who want to enhance and advance their practice by using ROM and feedback methods, but may not have the time or the resources to invest money or time into these methods. We have therefore pitched the content that follows at the no- and lo-tech end of the range but at the same time being informed by more advanced work.

In considering session-by-session change, there are several simple statistics that are helpful to all therapists. The first is the concept of *reliable change* – that is, change that can reasonably be attributed to the impact of therapy rather than measurement error (i.e., the inevitable error that is intrinsic to all measures, although some more than others). Reliable change addresses the question: how much has a patient's score changed and is it reliable? The extent of measurement error is measure-specific, so it is important to know what the *reliable change index* (RCI) is for the measure being used.

There is a view that the RCI is specific to the sample under investigation and therefore that the RCI needs to be calculated for each specific sample. The formulae for calculating the RCI is detailed in several journal articles (see Evans et al., 1998; Jacobson & Truax, 1991). However, pragmatically, with reports citing the RCI value using large samples of patients, it is reasonable to adopt reported values, as this also provides a better basis for making cross-study comparisons rather than each study generating its own value. The specific component of the RCI that is noteworthy is that it sets the level of improvement necessary for the change to be unlikely accountable by measurement error. Because the RCI is based on the psychometric properties of the specific measure being used, the value of the RCI is the same for all patients (in a specific sample or more generally) using that measure, regardless of their baseline score. Table 6.1 sets out the RCI values for some commonly-used outcome measures.

However, for example if the RCI for a specific measure is five points, the clinical meaning of a change by this amount will be different for a patient scoring at the severe end of the scale compared with a patient who is scoring in the mild range. This perspective is captured more in another often-used metric that adopts a change of 50 per cent from baseline score whereby a very high score will have to reduce more to meet this criterion as compared with a moderate score. This criterion has been more widely adopted in psychiatry-based studies.

The second concept that is a component of meaningful (statistical) change focuses on the end-point score indicating a patient to be more likely classed as a member of a non-clinical rather than a clinical population. These end-point scores have been used in the literature to designate clinically significant change, or more usually *clinically significant improvement*, when the score falls below the specified threshold. However, note as in Table 6.1 that for the ORS, improvement is indicated by a higher rather than a lower score. These thresholds are synonymous with those for determining *caseness* (e.g., whether

Table 6.1 Reliable change indices for commonly-used routine outcome measures

Outcome measure	Reliable change index	Caseness threshold
PHQ-9	6	≥ 10
GAD-7	4	≥ 8
CORE-OM	5	≥ 10
CORE-10	6	≥ 11
OQ-45	14	≥ 63
ORS (PCOMS)	6	≤ 25

or not a person's current level of distress meets criteria for clinically significant symptoms – a 'clinical case').

A combination of clinical significance and reliable change has been used widely to make an informed classification of patient outcome. These have been integrated into some hi-tech solutions, but can also be easily applied in no-tech and lo-tech solutions:

- *Reliable deterioration*: an increase in severity of the RCI or more since the initial session (e.g., a patient who started with a score of 14 on the PHQ-9 and now has a score of 21).
- *No reliable change*: the difference between the current score and the start of treatment is less than the RCI in either direction.
- *Reliable improvement*: a decrease in severity compared to the initial score of the RCI or more, but the score is not under the caseness threshold (e.g., a patient starting with a score of 20 on the PHQ-9, who has a current score of 12).
- *Recovered (reliable and clinically significant improvement)*: a decrease in severity compared to the initial score of the RCI or more, and having started in the clinical population (above caseness threshold) and currently scoring in the non-clinical range (under caseness threshold).

Note that these definitions refer to outcome measures where a low score is a good outcome, whereas some instrument scores go in the other direction (e.g., ORS).

Observing patterns in data: Shapes of change

Profiling the course of change across time in the psychological therapies has been a major focus of research since the seminal work of Kenneth Howard and colleagues mapping the relationship between the number of sessions of therapy (i.e., the dose) and patient outcomes (i.e., the response), resulting in the dose–response curve (Howard et al., 1986). Essentially, the dose–response curve depicted a negatively accelerating curve with a greater extent of change occurring during early sessions and continuing but with diminishing additional gains occurring thereafter. However, these data were based only on pre-post treatment outcomes and subsequent work using sessional data indicated that the dose–response effect has been widely documented across multiple treatment settings and conditions, but the relationship between outcomes and treatment duration varies across patients as a function of factors such as baseline severity (e.g., see reviews by Beard & Delgadillo, 2019; Bone et al., 2021; Kadera et al., 1996).

Access to repeated measures opened up new insights in the field of psychotherapy. Theoretically, the number of forms or shapes that repeated data can generate is infinite, being a function of the number of data points collected and a patient's response at each administration of a measure. Since the late 1980s and early 1990s, researchers and therapists have increasingly been analysing datasets comprising continuous data, very much in the way that has been the tradition in single-case studies but using aggregated data from multiple patients. Researchers and therapists have been using increasingly advanced methods to make predictions about the *expected treatment response* (ETR) of patients in treatment. This latter work became crucial to the underpinning for much of the subsequent yield in relation to clinical feedback systems that is the focus of subsequent chapters. However, in this chapter, we focus primarily on the observational yield of repeated measurement and some of the key classes of response that can be observed in repeated data. This is important as these patterns of data are not the focus of more hi-tech administrations, where the focus is on providing a signal based on the ETR. Hence, the patterns that we present here are ones that all therapists might find useful.

Here we briefly list the most common patterns or classes of change and present graphs to show the various patterns. As was mentioned in the introduction of this chapter, in the current chapter we will focus primarily on improving patterns. In Chapter 7, we will go into more detail on deteriorating patterns. In the examples, we have used a hypothetical measure – named simply as Outcome Measure – which has a maximum possible score of 100 and to which we have assigned a reliable change index of 15 and a clinical caseness threshold of 30 as reference points. We have also used a standard example of eight sessions simply for illustrative purposes.

> Sometimes you don't realise you have made progress, but if you got something on the screen showing what your scores were and what they are it quantifies your progress. Being able to track back though is very useful.
> – Anonymous patient, UK

Trends

Probably the pattern of response that many therapists view as the archetypal or ideal outcome profile is that of steady improvement from the start to end of therapy. Session-by-session improvement may be monotonic (i.e., each session's score is an improvement on the previous one), resulting in a steady trend towards better psychological health. But the improvement may also not be monotonic, and there may be an occasional worsening in scores at some sessions. These provide an observational signal to the therapist to check back to the individual items to see what may be accounting for the elevation in overall score, crucially to see whether it is a general worsening of most items or only a few with pronounced elevated scores. However, a pattern that shows a clear trend towards improvement is one where the benefit of clinical feedback (i.e., in keeping therapy progress on track) is least demonstrated. In effect, it provides good news in terms of feedback and therefore no signal that requires remedial action or a change of direction. But feedback to the patient on their positive progress can certainly be communicated to them.

In contrast, a deteriorating trend needs to be identified and acted on, but the question becomes one of deciding when deterioration is more than mere

Figure 6.1 Improving trend

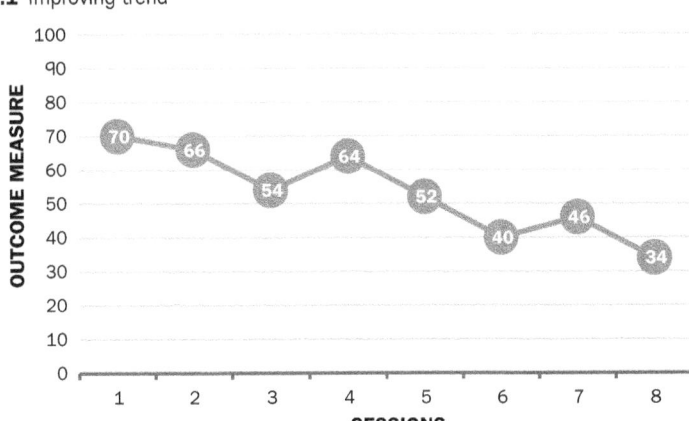

fluctuation in the measure (see Chapter 7). Some therapists may consider that any amount of deterioration is noteworthy and, at one level, this may be correct. But it is important to be mindful of measurement error; no measure is perfect and small fluctuations will occur. Information on how to act when a patient is deteriorating is discussed in detail in Chapter 8.

Early response

Another pattern of response that can be viewed as a form of trend is that of *early response*. The work on the dose–response effect highlighted the fact that a disproportionate percentage of improvement occurs in the initial sessions (Howard et al., 1986). This work can be viewed as the precursor to a focus on the phenomenon of early response whereby early gains within the first four sessions (defined as meeting the criterion of reliable improvement) are predictive of patients obtaining the subsequent status of reliable and clinically significant improvement at end of treatment (Beard & Delgadillo, 2019; Duffy et al., 2022). Although the duration of early response is broadly agreed as being four weeks, the criterion in relation to the change in measure varies as a function of the differing reliable change index (RCI) for the primary outcome measure (see Table 6.1).

Break points and sudden changes (sudden gains; sudden losses)

A second class of response pattern can be characterized by some form of break point in the data, namely a dramatic or sudden change in direction. In the literature, this is often referred to as a 'sudden gain' or a 'sudden loss'. The research literature has devised various criteria in order for the change in outcome measure to be termed a sudden gain or loss. However, before briefly outlining these, the first criterion is simply seeing in the data a change that is sudden (i.e., from

Figure 6.2 Improving trend with early response during the initial four sessions

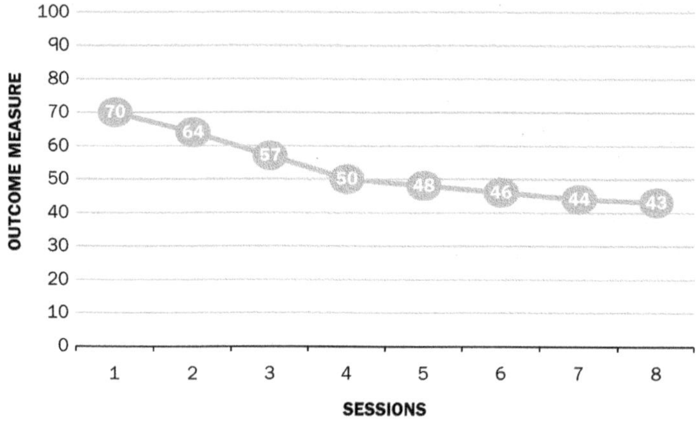

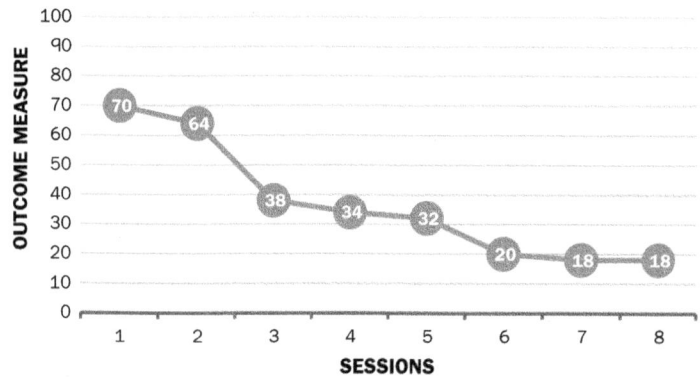

Figure 6.3 Break point exemplified by sudden gain between sessions 2 and 3

the data on one session to the next) and then of a magnitude that is clearly observable (i.e., that catches the eye if it is graphed). Figure 6.3 presents data that shows a sudden change (improvement) between sessions 2 and 3. But does it meet the criteria set out in the literature?

The definitions of sudden gains (and losses) require data to be stable for 2–3 sessions previously and then for the subsequent gain or loss to be maintained for 2–3 sessions. The reasoning here is that these criteria make it a more stringent threshold that indicates a significant shift from one state to another for the patient. Hence, for a therapist working in routine practice, a break point occurring at the second session would be of interest clinically but would not meet the criteria for a sudden gain in the research literature. Similarly, such a gain or loss that was not maintained would also be noteworthy to a therapist providing the extent of change was equal to or exceeded the reliable change index of the outcome measure.

The response of the therapist would be to show the feedback to the patient and use this as a starting point for discussing what has changed and to look at whether the change is reflected across a majority of items or whether it is a function of specific items. Of course, there are always life events that can have major impacts on the lives (and scores) of patients that include positive events (e.g., resolution of relationship issues, gaining employment) and negative events (e.g., the breakup of a significant relationship, loss of a loved one, loss of employment).

The phenomenon of sudden gains is defined by three criteria: (a) a reduction of points on the scale that is akin to the Reliable Change Index (i.e., the gain is large in absolute terms); (b) the reduction is equal to or more than 25 per cent of the preceding score (i.e., the reduction is large in relative terms); and (c) a significant difference on an independent t-test comparing the mean score for the three preceding sessions with the mean score for the three post-gain sessions (i.e., the gain is stable).

Two features are important to note in relation to sudden gains. First, like early response, sudden gains can predict final outcomes of therapy for a significant portion of patients (Shalom & Aderka, 2020). The fact that sudden gains tend to occur more often early on in the course of therapy makes them a useful signal for a good outcome. However, for a number of patients, these sudden gains are subsequently lost. Hence, sudden gain is not a guarantee of a positive final outcome. The second feature concerns an observation that has been made, namely that a sudden gain is just an extreme example of variability within a patient's score. In other words, as mentioned earlier, one pattern of response in data that can be seen in some patients' data is increasing degrees of variability and sudden gains are a pronounced form of variability. Patients can also have a combination of sudden gains and sudden losses (Lutz et al., 2013). Sudden losses are discussed in more detail in Chapter 7.

> It is often in key sessions where you see the penny drop and the ker-chunk moment and that is when the next week, you may see a shift in scores and that is when you can say something has really worked in that session and ask the patient: 'What was it about that session that was helpful? What have you done that is different that has made the difference?'
>
> – Anonymous therapist, UK

Turning points (curvilinear patterns; non-linear patterns)

The patterns discussed so far have all comprised overall straight lines or phases within the course of therapy that are visually straight. A further pattern that can comprise either straight or curved lines is where the data forms a V or U shape, or in this instance, an inverted V or U shape. In the inverted V shape, deterioration suddenly stops and the data starts on an improving course. In the U shape, the pattern is less discernible or dramatic and the changes between sessions may be relatively slight but graphing the data will

Figure 6.4 Turning point exemplifying improvement from session five onwards

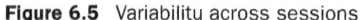

Figure 6.5 Variability across sessions

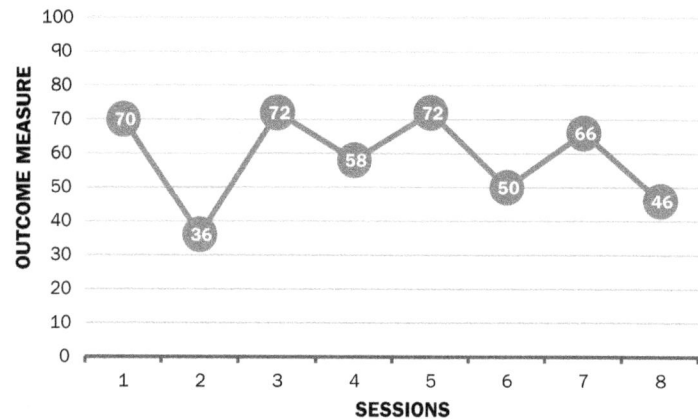

show that after a steady deterioration, the data turns a corner and gradually starts on an improving trajectory.

Variability (fluctuation intensity, instability)

In contrast to profiles that show trends in one direction or the other, some ROM profiles reflect substantial variability over the course of therapy – that is, they appear to have no clear direction but comprise a continuous alternating between improvement and deterioration, reflecting the ups and downs of daily life. It is often difficult to determine an overall picture of trend – it might be slightly improving but this is totally masked by the striking variability between the data points and where the aim of therapy will be to reduce the extent of variability.

Figure 6.6 Stability across sessions

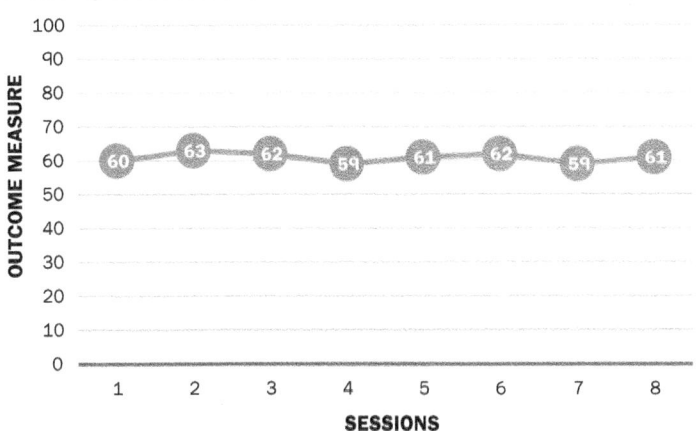

SESSIONS

Stability (no reliable change)

All the above patterns or classes of change have one feature in common, namely that they all show change in one direction or the other. In contrast to all these is a pattern where there is no change that can be considered reliable. The data profile for these patients can best be described as stable – that is, non-changing regardless of the actual severity level (see Figure 6.6). In such cases, the earlier session data (i.e., across the initial five sessions) is highly predictive of subsequent session scores. Research suggests that there is a substantial group of patients with a stable course (Lutz et al., 2014).

With such a pattern of data by session 5, it will be for the therapist to consider whether a change in the treatment delivery is appropriate. This might entail stepping up to a more intensive form of intervention if therapy is being delivered within a stepped care model (i.e., IAPT). Crucially, however, it warrants a discussion with the patient as to why the data shows little, if any, change. It should be mentioned that for a small percentage of patients, stabilizing them might be the best feasible outcome, whereas for others, a change in approach can shift their treatment trajectory substantially.

In all of the change patterns discussed in this chapter, it is important to discuss with the patient how they view the data, as there are three sources of information in the therapy room: the data, the therapist and the patient. It may be that the patient feels the therapy is helping them but is not reflected in the measure being used. It may be that therapy itself is helping them in not getting worse. In any event, it is likely that discussing the situation opening within the context of the therapeutic relationship will lead to a course of action that moves the patient on in one way or another (see Chapter 7 and 8).

On some of my recorded scores it did not look as if I had improved much, but I think that at the first session I had, I had gotten so used to feeling so low, that I had almost normalized it. I think when I very first filled one of the questionnaires in, I was almost in denial. I got so used to feeling rubbish, that it was only near the end of therapy, that I realised that some of my scores that had put down initially were just unrealistic.

– Anonymous patient, UK

Conclusions

This chapter has shown how the collection and plotting of patient data can provide the therapist, and patient, about progress that can then be used to aid decision-making about the course of therapy. The quote at the heading of the chapter asks therapists to look at the data before analysing it and this is our recommendation, namely for data to be used on a par with clinical experience. But, as we have stated, data can be over-interpreted and it is then important to apply the guidance regarding how much change is reliable, which again makes the point about how important it is to know the characteristics and features of the measure that is being used.

Key points in this chapter

- Being familiar with the specific values of the reliable change index and caseness for the outcome measure is essential.
- Engaging patients with the outcome from the initial session is crucial in giving the message that completing it and using the information is an important component of therapy.
- The number of patterns shown by the data are numerous but the main classes can be summarized as follows:
  - Trends (improving or deteriorating)
  - Early response (in the initial four sessions)
  - Break points (indicating sudden gains or losses)
  - Turning point (sustained change in direction)
  - Variability (alternating ups and downs)
  - Stability (no overall improvement or deterioration).

7 Recognizing when a patient is not improving

In this chapter

As discussed in Chapter 1, about 30–40 per cent of patients do not experience sufficient symptom reduction to be considered improved or recovered during psychological treatment, and for 5–10 per cent of patients their symptoms significantly worsen during treatment (De Jong, 2016; Wakefield et al., 2021). In this context, one of the main aims of using ROM and feedback is to prevent negative treatment outcomes, by adapting the treatment when feedback indicates that the patient is not progressing as well as might be expected. In this chapter, we explore response patterns that are associated with negative treatment outcomes. In addition, we discuss how you determine if your patient is making sufficient progress and how to have a conversation about it with the patient. In Chapter 8, we will present a model to formulate hypotheses about what is going on in the treatment and how to act upon that.

Unfavourable treatment response patterns

In Chapter 6, we presented a number of response patterns that can be observed when monitoring treatment outcomes. In this chapter, we will focus on response patterns that are associated with negative treatment outcomes. In the feedback literature, patients who are not progressing well in treatment are referred to as *not-on-track* (NOT) cases (Lambert, 2007) or *signal cases*, after the signal that some feedback systems provide when a patient does not progress sufficiently. Treatment can be classed as NOT for a variety of reasons (see Chapter 8), and as a result, there are an infinite number of potential response patterns. Yet, there are some patterns that occur more regularly, which are worth discussing in more detail.

> It shocked me when I had a dip in scores in the middle of my treatment, but we analysed what we thought what it was about, and that was useful.
> – Anonymous patient, UK

Negative trend

In some cases, outcome measure scores (e.g., representing symptom severity, functional impairment) gradually and slowly creep up. In Figure 7.1 you can see that there are no big increases over time, but yet the score of the outcome

Figure 7.1 Negative trend

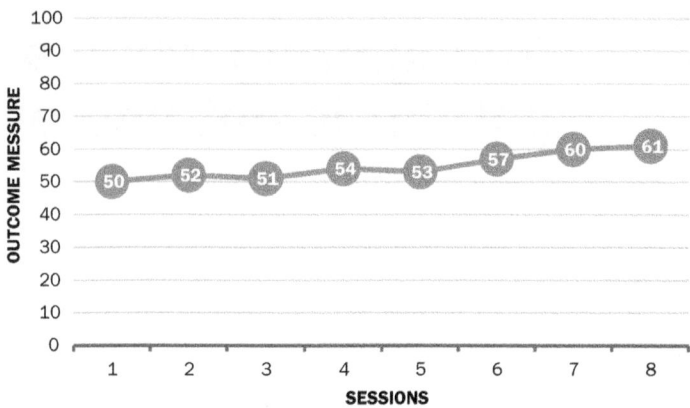

measure gradually increases to the point that there is more than a 20 per cent increase compared to the baseline at session 8. These trends are hard to notice, since the patient will seem to stay more or less the same, and thus it takes a while to notice that this might be more than just a bit of natural variation.

Sudden loss

A sudden loss indicates a worsening in functioning that (1) is large in absolute terms; (2) constitutes a worsening in scores of 25 per cent or more; and (3) remains stable in the sessions after the loss occurs. Sudden losses are the opposite of sudden gains (see Chapter 6), a concept developed by Tang and DeRubeis (1999) that has been substantially studied in psychotherapy. A recent meta-analysis found that sudden gains significantly predict treatment outcomes across a variety of treatments, disorders and settings (Shalom & Aderka, 2020). However, sudden losses are not commonly reported in most studies, and as a result we know less about their predictive value. One large study looking at 1500 treatment trajectories assessed the effect of sudden gains and sudden losses on treatment outcomes (Lutz et al., 2013). The results indicated that both sudden gains and sudden losses (and their combination) predict treatment outcomes. Patients with sudden gains (improvements) experienced substantially more symptom reduction, fewer interpersonal problems, and better emotional well-being compared to other patients. Patients with sudden losses (deterioration) had substantially more symptoms and interpersonal problems and lower levels of emotional well-being compared to other patients, which indicates that sudden losses have a higher probability of negative treatment results. Patients with sudden gains also rated the therapeutic relationship significantly more positive for that session than patients in sudden loss sessions (Lutz et al., 2013). Thus, if a patient experiences a sudden loss, it is important to act upon it. The results regarding the therapeutic relationship ratings suggests that a problematic

Figure 7.2 Sudden loss

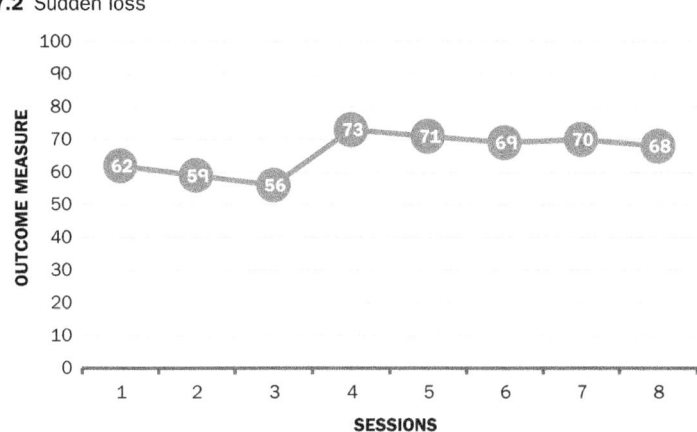

relationship might be a risk factor for sudden losses. An example of a sudden loss is presented in Figure 7.2.

No change

A stable pattern in scores can be a good thing (see Chapter 6), but it can also be an indication of a poor treatment response. In Figure 7.3 an example of a case with persistently severe symptoms is presented. As can be seen, there is some degree of natural fluctuation, but overall there does not seem to be any substantial improvements. In patients with a high severity level you would normally expect to see change, since there is a lot of room for improvement (i.e., regression to the mean). However, research on change patterns indicates that a subgroup of patients (approximately 20 per cent) shows a pattern of stable symptom levels that continues to be high throughout treatment. While these patients do not improve in symptoms, they do experience improvements in psychological well-being and life-functioning (i.e., Stulz & Lutz, 2007). This could be an indication to assess different domains in these patients, for example when patients might have more chronic and severe psychological problems (e.g., psychotic disorder) that may not necessarily be expected to improve, but where things like a better functioning in life or a better quality of life could be obtainable.

If no change occurs in a patient who had low symptom severity at the start of treatment, then something else might be the case. See for example Figure 7.4., in which the patient starts relatively close to the cut-off of normal functioning (30 for this hypothetical measure). This low score could be due to several reasons, such as the selected outcome measure not capturing the symptoms that the patient experiences (e.g., eating disorders, autism spectrum disorder) or the patient seeking treatment for other reasons than symptom reduction (e.g., couples counselling). Alternatively, the lack of change could be an indication that the treatment is not working well for the patient.

Figure 7.3 No change, high severity

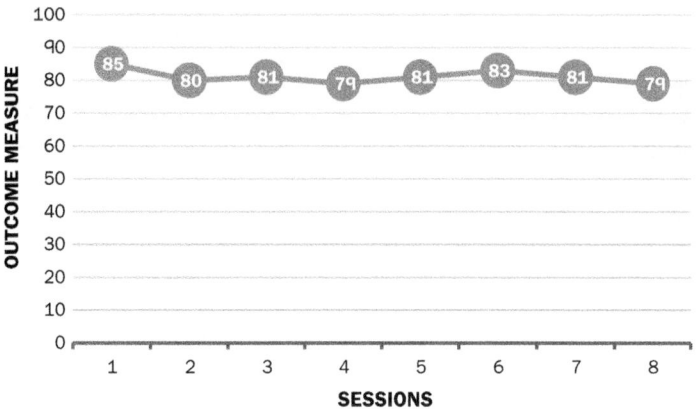

Figure 7.4 No change, low severity

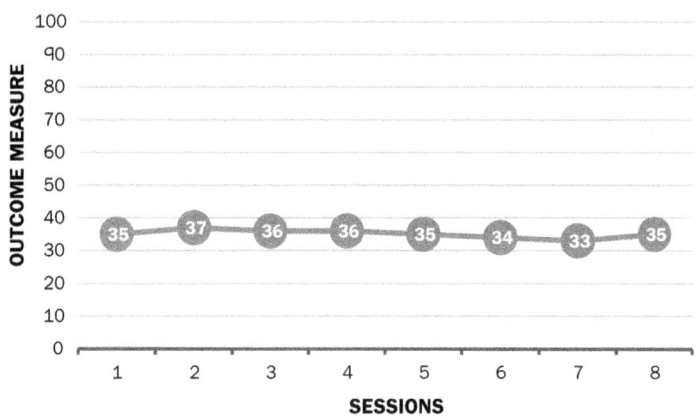

Negative turning point

In some cases, an initial improvement is observed, but after a couple of sessions the patient experiences a worsening in symptoms (see Figure 7.5). The curves in this case show a V shape (sharp change) or a U shape (more gradual change). Anecdotally, there are some potential causes for this pattern: (1) the patient gains insight in their symptoms during treatment and starts to become more aware of them; (2) the patient is high in avoidance and due to the therapy needs to start talking about painful topics (e.g., trauma) more or needs to start practising behaviour they have been avoiding (e.g., social interactions); and (3) the patient is triggered by something during the treatment, but does not know how to bring it up with the therapist. For the first two reasons, a temporary increase in symptoms might be an indication that the therapy might still have a potential to work. However, it is important to mention that this pattern

Figure 7.5 Negative turning point in session 4, after which the outcomes deteriorate

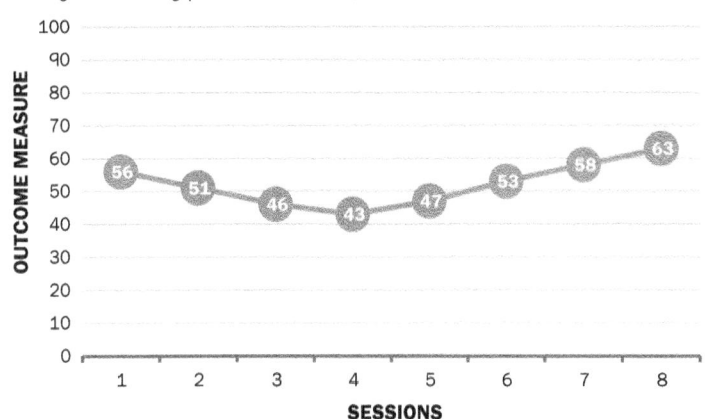

Figure 7.6 High variability in a patient with a relatively high severity

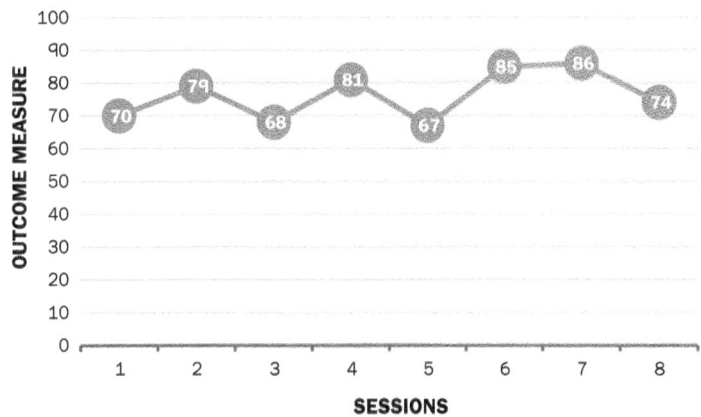

is atypical for successful treatment, and ultimately the outcomes need to improve again in a few sessions. For the third reason, there might be a problem in the therapeutic alliance that might be worth exploring (see more on that in Chapter 8).

High variability

Some patients show a pattern of variability, for example a combination of sudden gains and sudden losses in symptom distress (see Figure 7.6 for an example). This high variability is typically an indication for a risk of negative treatment outcomes (Lutz et al., 2013). For some patients this variability is caused by a lack of emotion regulation skills (e.g., patients with borderline personality disorder), while for others there may be an unstable situation in life (e.g., dealing with severe adversities).

How much change is enough?

A case is classified as *not-on-track* (NOT) when, at a certain point in treatment, a substantial worsening of symptoms is evident. And you may wonder: 'Why is it so important to identify that a patient is not progressing as expected at one moment in treatment? Maybe they are just having a bad week.' Of course, that can certainly be the case. However, we know from scientific research that when a patient experiences a significant worsening of symptoms, that even one such week increases the chances of their ending treatment either unchanged or worsened. Lutz and colleagues (2006) found that patients who deviated from an expected treatment course just once had over a 50 per cent chance – 53 per cent to be precise – of ending treatment with a negative outcome, compared to 30 per cent of patients who did not yield such a signal during treatment. Moreover, if a patient's ROM scores provided a signal twice over the course of treatment, the odds of a negative outcome increased to 70 per cent, while patients who had three or more signals had a 74 per cent chance of ending treatment with negative outcomes. This shows that even a single week of worsening symptoms is important to pay attention to, as it already strongly increases the odds of ending treatment with unfavourable results.

Now, how do we decide whether an increase in symptoms is clinically important? Larger changes in symptoms might be easy to observe, but smaller changes can be harder to detect. This is further complicated by the fact that every measurement contains measurement error. Hence, a small difference between two scores might not be a true change in symptoms, but rather an artefact of the measurement error of the instrument. So how do we know whether the difference between two scores is a real difference? Research tells us that when people experience an event as negative, they have a tendency to attribute the information to external factors (e.g., another person, or circumstances). In the same way, therapists often try to reason away why there is a worsening of symptoms (e.g., the patient has a higher symptom level because 'sometimes patients get worse before they get better'). Similarly, it might be tempting to rationalize away a patient's worsening scores based on the myth that there is no gain without pain. As a safeguard, therefore, it is recommended to use pre-set criteria to determine when you need to act on the feedback, so that such biases can be avoided.

In general, there are two major approaches when it comes to determining if there is sufficient progress: the rational and the empirical method. We address each of these in turn.

Rational methods

When you start using a feedback system, there is often no available data on how patients in your particular mental health care setting typically respond to treatment. In these cases, it can be useful to use a rational method of determining when a patient is considered to be *not-on-track*. The rational method determines a cut-off point for considering a case to have worsened based on a rationally-derived statistical rules. Fortunately, rational methods are performing relatively well, compared to empirical methods (Lutz et al., 2006). There are several approaches or rules that can be used, in part depending on the information that is available about the outcome instrument and we describe three such approaches: clinical rule of thumb, distribution-based rule, and psychometric rule.

Clinical rule of thumb: This method uses a criterion related to the performance of the outcome measure being used that is based on clinical impressions. For instance, for the Outcome Rating Scale (ORS; Miller et al., 2003) a rule of thumb that is sometimes used comprises a five-point improvement to be achieved within the first five sessions of therapy. There are also empirical methods available for the ORS but the clinical rule of thumb is based on reasoning that research shows that the largest amount of change happens in the earlier stages of therapy. Hence, if there does not seem to be progress by the end of those initial five sessions, then it might be time to change therapist or treatment strategy. While the rule is, to some degree, arbitrary, it seems reasonable from a clinical point of view, is more actionable than visual inspection of data, and it is easy to remember (five points over five sessions). The disadvantage of this method is that it is not informed by data, which may lead it to be somewhat crude. However, it should be said that some rules work rather well and this method is likely to do better than clinical judgement alone. In this particular example, the rule might work less well with patients starting treatment in the lower severity range, who have less room for improvement and for whom a five-point decrease in symptoms might be harder to achieve.

Distribution-based rule: Some systems use a distribution-based rule, usually based on the population norms for an instrument. Based on the distribution of scores for a measure, you could argue that a certain percentile corresponds with a certain risk. For instance, one of the graphs displayed in the NORSE system (Hovland & Moltu, 2019) highlights the severity of symptoms based on certain percentiles. In Figure 7.7 an example for such a system is provided. As you can see, black is used for very high scores that are above the 90th percentile (depressive symptoms), dark grey if they are in the 80–90th percentile range (interpersonal problems), light grey in the 50–80th percentile range (anxiety), and white for scores below the 50th percentile (somatic). The advantage of this system is that high scores are objectively high, and are easy to interpret: '90 per cent of patients score lower than this patient on this scale'.

The limitation of such systems as these is that they do not take change into account. Rather, they record successive high scores in isolation rather than in relation to any previous score. So, if a patient starts in a very high percentile, for instance the 94th percentile, and improves a fair amount and at the second measurement is at the 81st percentile, they would still be marked as high even though they have improved relative to their previous score. Feeding back such information may be demotivating for the patient and it is then the task of the therapist in such cases to point out the change that has already been achieved.

Psychometric rule: This method uses certain psychometric properties or characteristics of the outcome instrument as a criterion. For example, a common method in ROM systems is to take the *reliable change index* (RCI) of an instrument and use it to determine whether a patient has worsened. The reliable

Figure 7.7 Example of applying a distribution-based rule

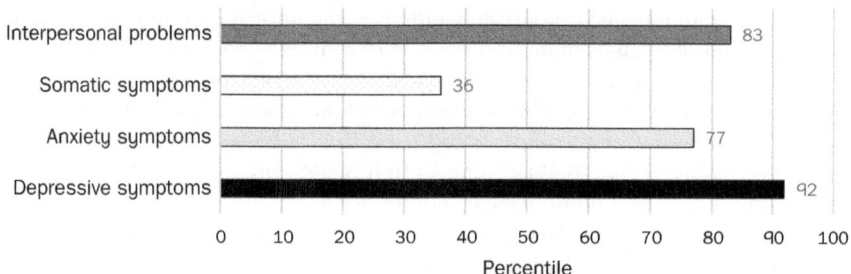

change index is a characteristic of a measurement instrument that represents the magnitude of change that is needed to be certain that changes are not simply explained by measurement error or chance. The calculation is based on the reliability of the measure (Jacobson & Truax, 1991). In short, the more reliable a measure is, the smaller the measurement error will be. So, it can be seen that not all measures will yield the same measurement error and one of the attractions of the RCI is that the index is specific to a given measure. Hence, it is important to use validated outcome measures with good reliability properties (e.g., high indices of internal consistency, test–retest reliability).

So, returning to the use of the RCI, if a patient worsens by the amount of the RCI or more on an instrument, they are considered to have deteriorated. For instance, the Outcome Questionnaire-45 (Lambert et al., 2004) has an RCI of 14 points. So, if a patient's score increases by 14 points compared to their intake score, they would be considered to be *not-on-track*. An example of such a method is provided in Figure 7.8. The patient has an initial score of 84, and if they worsen by 14 points to a score of 98 (the grey dotted line) they would be considered *not-on-track*. In the example, the patient is not-on-track at measurement 3. While this method is intuitively appealing, in practice the RCI requires a fairly large change, which is useful for evaluating the final result of therapy, but is less useful to evaluate progress during therapy. Of course, if a patient classifies as deteriorated during treatment, it should be taken seriously, but smaller amounts of worsening of symptoms are likely also to be relevant. An alternative to the RCI could be to use the raw measurement error of the instrument, which is typically smaller than the RCI. For example, in case of the OQ-45, the measurement error is 6.8, which would then require a patient to worsen 7 points in order to be classified as *not-on-track*.

Empirical methods

In contrast to rational approaches, empirical methods use data from patients who have been in treatment earlier and use a database to create so-called *expected treatment response* (ETR) curves. ETR curves are developed using session-by-session outcome data from large groups of patients who have been treated in a similar setting. These data are used to predict how new patients with similar characteristics (e.g., similar initial symptom severity) will progress

Figure 7.8 Example of psychometric rule using the reliable change index (RCI)

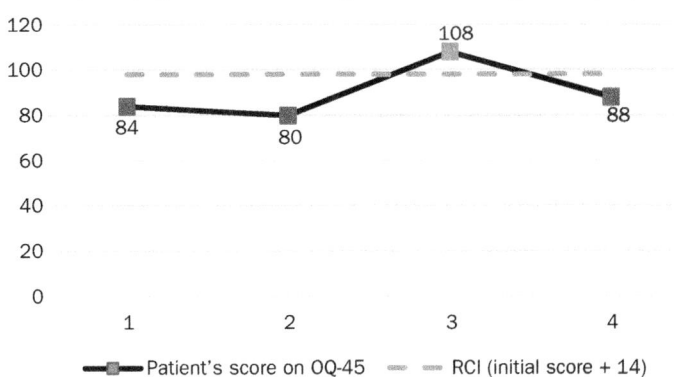

Figure 7.9 Example of a not-on-track case using the empirical ETR method

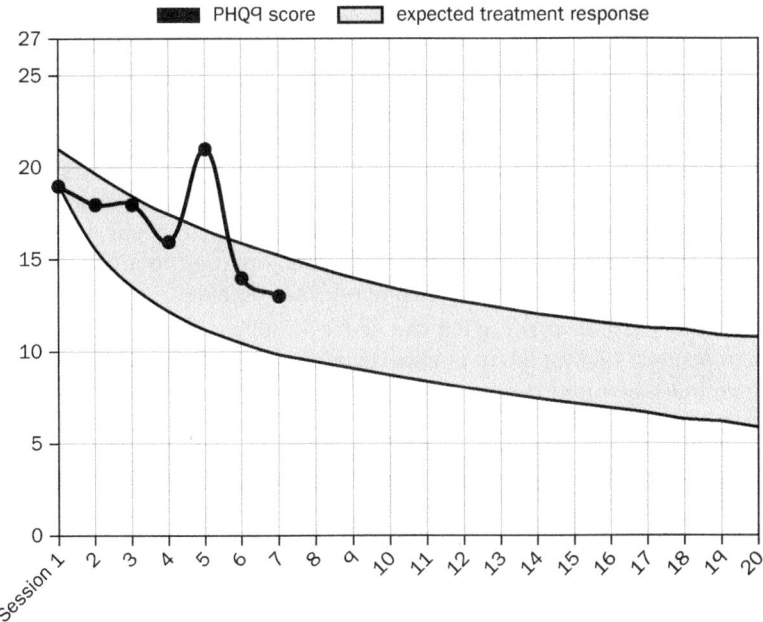

in therapy. During treatment, a patient's actual progress can be compared with the prediction from the ETR curve and, when someone deviates too much from the predicted course, a warning signal is given to the therapist that the patient is not-on-track. In Figure 7.9, the ETR curve, and the surrounding confidence intervals, are visualized by the grey zone. As long as the patient's measures are in the grey zone, the treatment is considered to be on track. However, at the 5th measurement, the patient scores above the upper or 'failure boundary' of the ETR curve, and the treatment is considered to be not-on-track.

Discussing the feedback with the patient

Many therapists find discussing a lack of progress with a patient uncomfortable. Of course, the message that the patient is showing a worsening in symptoms is not always a pleasant message to give, but it is good to remember that the patient most likely is aware of the severity of symptoms they are experiencing. After all, they completed the questionnaires themselves and know that they have not been feeling well. Also, as we will discuss later in this chapter, there are multiple possibilities for why a patient is not progressing well. Importantly, it does not necessarily mean that the treatment is failing. Indeed, it is crucial to avoid terminology such as 'failing' and 'failure'. One of the key axioms of working with data is that we learn from it and what comes from it is a learning experience.

In order to guide your thinking and actions, the following questions might prove useful:

- **Does the patient recognize the score?** Sometimes there is a discrepancy between the score and how the patient is feeling. For instance, a patient may say, 'I'm doing ok this week,' but scores in the 70th percentile. In that case, it could be good to discuss this apparent discrepancy with the patient. Another situation that could occur is that the instrument does not capture everything that you are working on in therapy. So perhaps the patient has experienced a lot of change in one particular area, but less so in other areas that are measured by the instrument. This situation is more likely to occur when a single and narrowly specific measure is applied, as opposed to a combination of measures that capture more than one relevant domain.

- **Does the patient agree with the score?** Suppose the scales of an instrument suggest that a patient is experiencing a lot of distress in social situations, but when you raise this with them, the patient disagrees with it. In these cases, it is also helpful to discuss with the patient what might be causing the discrepancy. Importantly, it is not the aim to find out which perspective is correct but rather for the discussion to lead to learning something about the experience.

- **How does the patient feel about the amount of change that has been made so far?** If there is a deterioration in symptoms, it is likely that the patient will be disappointed with that, but sometimes it is the best that can be achieved at a certain point in time. Also, in some cases, patients have gained an increased understanding of their symptoms, causing them to increase in score (i.e., worsen), although it should be mentioned that this is a less typical pattern of change.

- **Does something need to change?** It may not be necessary to change the treatment plan in all NOT cases, but it is important to openly discuss this option with the patient, as it gives the signal to the patient that you are open to their (verbal) feedback. Many patients find it hard to discuss that they are not happy with how therapy is going.

In Box 7.1 is one example of how a feedback conversation might proceed.

Box 7.1 A feedback conversation

T: Let's have a look at your progress chart. This line here is the progress you have made over time. This (points at start of treatment) is where we started, and this (points at last measurement) is where we are now. Your score right now tells us that you are experiencing substantial distress, and that this has even increased since the start of treatment. Does this fit with how you have been feeling this week?

P: Well, I have been feeling pretty down in the last week. I have not been sleeping well, and it has been really tough even getting out of bed in the morning.

T: I'm sorry to hear that. Do you think the lack of sleep is what has been causing you to feel down, or are there also other things that might be useful to take into account?

P: Well, the lack of sleep has definitely contributed, but...

T: Anything else?

P: Um... I've been worrying a lot lately, especially when I'm in bed. So when I wake up at night to go to the bathroom, my head is 'on' immediately, and I start thinking about the situation at work, and then I can't sleep anymore for hours, until, like, 5 a.m., when I doze off again, because I feel exhausted.

T: So, do you feel that this has been causing you to feel down?

P: Yeah...

T: Apart from the situation at work, how do you feel the therapy is working for you? Is there something I could be doing differently, for example? In order to help you in a better way...

P: Uhm... no not right now.

T: If at some point in the therapy you do feel like there is something you would like to change, do let me know. I am not perfect, and it is important to me that we could talk about it, if I were to do something you do not like. That way we can talk about how to do things differently.

P: Ok. I will.

T: Thank you. Now let's get back to discussing this situation at work, which seems to be making things pretty difficult.

During the training, we practised what to say to patients when they were worsening. We discussed that it is helpful to refrain from using phrases like 'you are doing bad' or 'you are moving in the wrong direction', but rather use phrases like 'let's look at your symptoms; it looks like they are changing'. Our fear was that it might otherwise come across to the patient as if they were failing.

– Anonymous therapist, UK

The first thing you say after you get feedback from the client is going to either reinforce or punish what was said. So, I think it is critical how we model receptiveness. And it can be pretty hard for me. I know that those moments where I feel like I have tried the hardest and strained to the most to reach beyond my abilities. And then I get some piece of negative feedback. Even after 22 years of doing it, it stings.

– Scott Miller, feedback system developer and trainer, USA

Conclusions

In routine practice, a substantial number of cases show a lack of progress or even worsening in symptoms or functioning at some point in their treatment. As a result, all therapists will encounter this from time to time, and addressing this with the patient might be uncomfortable. It is important to realize that, as therapists, we cannot help everyone. On average 30–50 per cent of patients will not benefit from treatment in routine care, so it is important to master the skill of dealing with this in therapy. Of course, without ROM and feedback, you would also have patients who do not improve, but the ROM will make it very explicit and visible. In this chapter, we have presented methods to help you identify when a treatment is not progressing well, and the type of pattern the patient displays may even tell you something about what might be going on. The next step is to then discuss the results of the ROM and feedback with the patient. In the next chapter, we will discuss more elaborately how to adapt the case formulation and treatment plan (if necessary) in NOT cases.

Key points in this chapter

- Certain change patterns indicate that therapy is not working well and the patient may be at risk of a poor treatment outcome. Cases showing these patterns are referred to as *not-on-track* (NOT).
- There are different ways to determine when treatment is NOT and therapists can use rational methods or empirical methods.
- The method to use depends upon how much data has already been collected on the feedback instrument, as some methods require large volumes of data to generate empirical decision-rules.
- Obtain the patient's perspective on whether they think the change they have made up until that point in therapy seems accurate to them and seems good enough or not.

8 Clinical troubleshooting for non-improving patients

In this chapter

In Chapter 7, we have discussed how to recognize *when* therapy is not progressing well. In the current chapter, we are diving deeper into determining *what* you can do when your patient is displaying a lack of progress. We will provide an evidence-based model to identify and to deal with common challenges that get in the way of effective therapy. We conclude with suggestions about how to discuss progress feedback with your patient and how you can troubleshoot collaboratively to adapt treatment in order to improve treatment outcomes.

Basic principles of clinical troubleshooting

As discussed in previous chapters, feedback technology was designed to identify cases that are not progressing as well as we might expect. This serves a practical goal, which is to identify and rectify problems that might be interfering with treatment progress. Thus, feedback-informed treatment has two linked processes: (1) the identification of NOT cases; and (2) the clinical actions and decisions that follow. The first is a classification process, and it relies on the interpretation of routine outcome measures. Such a classification process can be achieved using decision rules and/or statistical models, as discussed in Chapter 7. The second is a clinical process, which ultimately aims to identify and deal with problems that come up during therapy, and for this reason we refer to it as *clinical troubleshooting*. This troubleshooting process is based on a number of assumptions that are grounded in the empirical literature that is covered in earlier chapters of this book. The key assumptions are summarized below:

- Different patients respond differently to psychotherapy. Some patients are more likely than others to improve during therapy.
- NOT signals help us to identify patients who may not attain symptomatic improvement and patients who might actually be on a trajectory of deterioration.
- NOT signals are not completely random; they can be explained by a range of factors that are described below.

- There is no single or simple explanation for a NOT signal. NOT signals could be influenced by one or more factors. Some of these factors are amenable to change, whereas others are not.
- Adjusting the treatment plan based on the factors that are relevant to each patient can help to improve outcomes, or at least reduce the risk of deterioration.

Clinical troubleshooting involves acting on and making decisions that are based on the above assumptions. Furthermore, in our experience, effective trouble-shooting actions adhere to the following six principles (and that can be recalled using the mnemonic CCEEPP):

- **Curiosity:** Don't assume that you know why a patient is not responding well to therapy. Adopt a stance of curiosity, willingness to learn and openness to the possibility that your assumptions and intuitions could be inaccurate.
- **Collaboration:** Therapy requires teamwork to get the best possible result. If things aren't going so well, make sure that the patient and your clinical supervisor are closely involved in the troubleshooting plan.
- **Empiricism:** Effective troubleshooting is informed by research evidence on predictors of treatment progress in psychotherapy and evidence-based treatment strategies.
- **Experimentation:** Effective troubleshooting brings the scientific method into the treatment plan by forming a hypothesis about the NOT signal and formally testing this hypothesis through an experimental manipulation (a specific modification to the treatment plan). Routine outcome monitoring can then be used as data to support or to refute your hypothesis about the NOT signal and the effectiveness of your troubleshooting plan.
- **Personalization:** If therapy isn't going well, it is necessary to adjust it to the patient's unique circumstances and characteristics in order to make it more relevant, acceptable and effective.
- **Parsimony:** Don't overcomplicate things. Sometimes, simple solutions can help to deal with complicated problems. In general, you should favour a simple and plausible explanation rather than an overly complicated one.

The six steps of troubleshooting

We now outline a clinical troubleshooting method that is grounded in all of the above assumptions and principles, and which has been empirically tested in a large, multi-service randomized controlled trial (Delgadillo et al., 2018). This method can be broken down into six discrete steps (see Figure 8.1):

1 *Exploring* and identifying obstacles
2 *Generating* hypotheses and formulating obstacles
3 *Developing* a troubleshooting plan

4 *Implementing* a plan
5 *Evaluating*
6 *Reviewing* the overall treatment plan.

Step 1: Exploring and identifying clinically relevant factors

The first step involves exploring factors that might be relevant to treatment progress, with reference to three sources of information: (1) the empirical literature; (2) the patient's perspective; and (3) the perspective of your peers and/or clinical supervisor. This approach aims to achieve a balance between the principles of empiricism and collaboration. If treatment is NOT, you should start your exploration by considering whether one or more known prognostic indicators may be relevant to the specific case. Prognostic indicators are variables that are statistically associated with psychological treatment outcomes. The diagram shown in Figure 8.2 integrates several factors that have been examined in process–outcome studies of progress feedback (e.g., Probst et al., 2015, 2020; Schilling et al., 2021; White et al., 2015; Williams, 2021) and in studies investigating prognostic indicators of poor treatment response which are associated with NOT signals (e.g., Delgadillo et al., 2016). This model can be used as a useful framework to generate preliminary hypotheses. The model captures two layers of variables referred to as *risk factors* and *processes*. Risk factors are general prognostic indicators associated with heightened distress and a lower probability of full remission of symptoms. Processes refer to mechanisms through which the risk factors exert their influence on the treatment and

Figure 8.1 The six steps of clinical troubleshooting

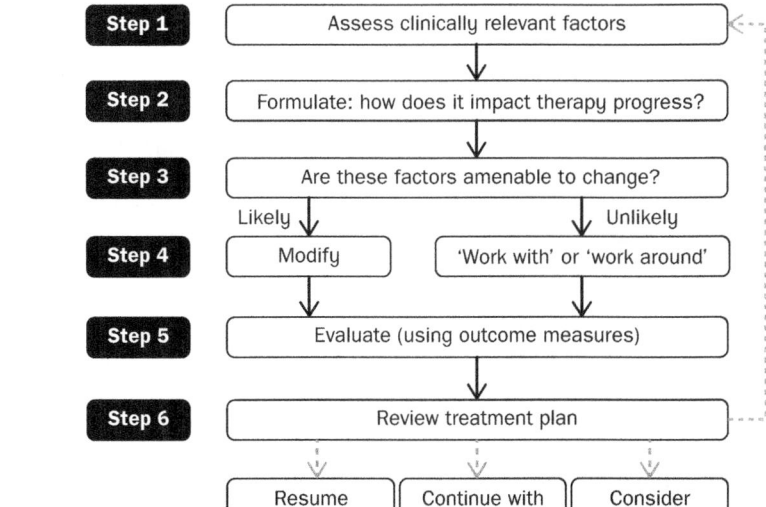

its chance of success or failure. For example, a patient with a history of adverse childhood adversity (e.g., neglect, abuse) may find it difficult to trust people, including the therapist, leading to an alliance deficit, which in turn can attenuate the effects of therapy. In another example, a patient's comorbid chronic health illness and disability may undermine their expectations of improvement in their mental health, in turn resulting in lower motivation to adhere to therapy tasks. In this way, we can use insights from the literature in the field of progress feedback to form initial hypotheses about why a patient's treatment may seem stuck or complicated.

For instance, a patient's panic disorder may be complicated by a comorbid chronic pain problem which limits their ability to walk and move, leading to considerable functional impairment in their management of daily tasks such as climbing stairs, carrying objects and walking long distances. This case is illustrative of prognostic risk factors (chronic pain, disability and functional impairment). Another patient's depression may be complicated by their constant sense of feeling misunderstood, racially discriminated and rejected by others, including their therapist, who happens to be going through a period of occupational burnout and general dissatisfaction with their work conditions. This second case includes relevant prognostic risk factors (minority stress) and process factors (alliance deficit).

In another case, Annie, a teenage college student who lives by herself in university dorms, experiences depression and social anxiety, complicated by the fact that she is not taking any practical steps to interact with people, despite her therapist's encouragements to do so, because she does not expect that this will work for her and therefore thinks there is little point in trying to connect with others. She finds it hard to get along with people and doesn't feel that she knows how to form and maintain relationships. Annie's case includes relevant risk factors (social isolation and interpersonal difficulties) and process factors (expectancy and motivational deficits). All three of these case vignettes illustrate factors depicted in Figure 8.2. In the rest of this chapter, we will refer to Annie's case as an illustrative example.

In order to identify relevant factors, this first step involves starting a dialogue with the patient once the NOT signal has been recognized, and formulating questions that explore each of the layers depicted in Figure 8.2. Box 8.1 provides an example of such a dialogue. The dialogue in Box 8.1 illustrates the principle of *curiosity* outlined above, whereby the therapist is open to the possibility that one or more factors may be relevant to Annie and the treatment process. This vignette exemplifies the use of open questions that aim to explore the factors in Figure 8.2; including prognostic risk factors (e.g., financial, relational problems) and therapy processes that can be directly worked on (e.g., alliance, expectancy, dealing with life events and problems). Annie's example illustrates an assessment process that starts by considering wider contextual factors and which moves towards more specific process and individual factors. In this case, the relevance of contextual factors was unclear, so the therapist continued to explore other factors. No obvious alliance ruptures were identified when the therapist explored Annie's views about the therapy process, but

Figure 8.2 Overview of prognostic risk factors and therapy processes that can influence a patient's treatment response

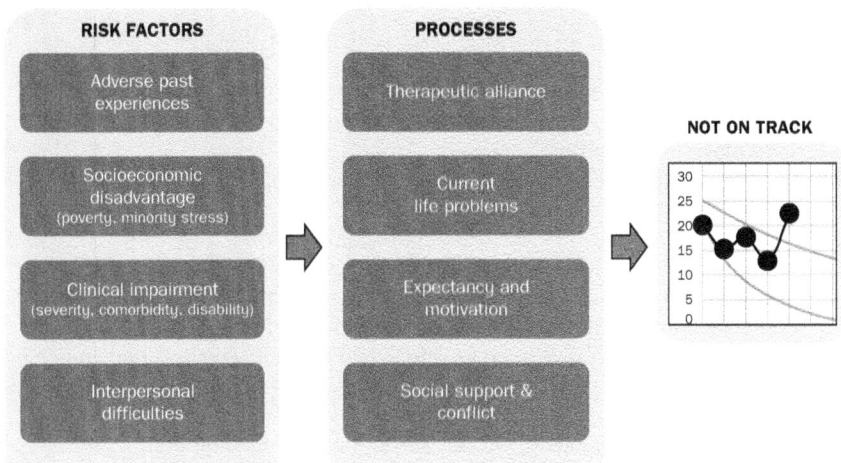

it was clear that she was struggling to adhere to therapy tasks that involved gradual restoration of social contact. Furthermore, the relevance of social isolation became more apparent, as well as the relevance of low expectations about the therapy tasks. In summary, Annie's case illustrates an interaction of individual risk factors (single/lonely) and process factors (homework non-adherence related to low expectancy, persistent negative thoughts and their emotional consequences).

This assessment process, starting with wider contextual factors (such as socioeconomic issues and life events) and moving towards individual patient factors (e.g., comorbidities, disability, interpersonal difficulties), is advisable for two reasons. Firstly, it is known that stressful life events are often implicated in the onset and maintenance of a variety of mental health problems and therefore constitute a plausible starting point for assessment. Similarly, there is a well-developed evidence base for the relevance of process factors such as those listed in Figure 8.2, which is why we tend to explore this area before considering patient-specific factors (e.g., see Norcross & Lambert, 2018). Secondly, this method encourages us not to jump to the conclusion that poor progress is necessarily explained by a patient's characteristics. Sometimes therapists automatically assume that lack of symptomatic improvement 'is the patient's fault' (e.g., not adhering to therapy tasks, resistant, unmotivated, not 'psychologically minded', invested in maintaining a 'sick role', etc.). The method described above is a good way to train ourselves to be open minded about the possible reasons for poor progress, while adopting a collaborative and empirical stance. This approach is also a good way to train ourselves to recognize that poor progress may be influenced by our own reactions and circumstances as therapists. Of course, a therapist may also choose to explore these factors in a different order if it seems most consistent with the patient's concerns.

Box 8.1 Exploring clinically relevant factors in Annie's case

T: According to today's progress chart, it seems that your depression symptoms have been getting more intense over the last week. What do you think? Does that fit with your experience?

P: Um... I guess so. I just feel awful all the time, no matter what I do to try to make things better.

T: That sounds really upsetting. I wonder if we could try to figure out why things continue to feel so difficult.

P: OK.

T: Sometimes people feel stuck with these feelings of depression because difficult life events continue to make things hard. Can you think of any recent events that may have made things more difficult?

P: Um, I don't know... I've been mostly in bed all week, I haven't done much at all.

T: Oh.

P: Yeah, I feel really lonely, but terrified of being around others.

T: I get it. It's very hard to face people and activities when your symptoms are so severe, and that's making you feel quite isolated. So, if your symptoms haven't been made worse by any recent events, what about problems that could be a constant source of stress, such as financial problems or relationship problems?

P: I don't think so. My family helps me to pay bills and stuff while I try to finish my college degree.

T: I see...

P: I get along OK with my family.

T: Right. So, it doesn't sound like there are any recent events, financial or relationship issues that might explain your recent increase in symptoms.

P: No, I don't think so.

T: Maybe there's another explanation. Sometimes people get worse if they don't feel that therapy is going very well or doesn't meet their expectations. I'm interested to know what you think about our sessions so far. How do you think it's going?

P: Um... I find it helpful to talk with you. I know we said that I would try to contact friends online again, but I just haven't felt able to do that lately, and I'm not really sure if that would help anyway...

For instance, the dialogue in Box 8.1 starts by acknowledging that symptoms are not on track, and then proceeds by exploring wider contextual factors (life events, finances, relationships) and process factors (alliance, expectancy). With experience, therapists can adapt their questioning style to be responsive to a patient's concerns and presentation, nevertheless exploring all of the factors depicted in Figure 8.2.

Some feedback systems include *clinical support tools*, which assess some of these factors automatically when a case is classified as NOT. For example, the OQ Analyst software launches an additional questionnaire named the Assessment for Signal Clients (ASC) that assesses four domains that are related to NOT

signals: the therapeutic alliance, the patient's motivation to change, social support deficits, and (coping with) stressful life events. The ASC has also been
incorporated in other feedback systems, in some cases supplemented with additional domains (e.g., Lucock et al., 2015; Lutz et al., 2019). Research suggests
that difficulties in alliance and motivation tend to co-occur in a substantial number of patients, as do difficulties in social support and (coping with) stressful life
events (White et al., 2015). A relatively large number of NOT cases had difficulties with social support, which perhaps makes the patient vulnerable in dealing
with stressful life events, as the therapist may be one of the few people the patient
has with whom they can talk about stressful events. Social support, life events
and motivation problems are often endorsed by NOT patients (Schilling et al.,
2021). Item-level analyses indicated that interpersonal difficulties outside of
therapy were associated with NOT signals (Probst et al., 2015, 2020).

A recent qualitative study assessed the case notes from 192 therapy sessions
classified as NOT and listed obstacles and solutions that were identified by
experienced feedback-using therapists (Williams, 2021). The obstacles that were
most commonly identified were related to distressing past experiences, attitudes and behaviours that interfered with treatment adherence, social network
related problems and stress, current stressors (e.g., financial stress) and therapy
factors (e.g., lack of agreement on goals and tasks of therapy). Furthermore,
the solutions that were identified included supporting tasks (e.g., modelling
and supporting patients to practise coping skills), focality (e.g., having a clear
focus for the therapy session), bridging (e.g., ensuring there is continuity in the
content covered from session-to-session) and using a personalized case formulation (which incorporates information about obstacles, such as described in
step 2 below). This research reveals that there are many possible obstacles that
can arise during treatment, and these can be highly idiographic (i.e., person-specific), which requires therapists to carefully assess various possible
domains (as described above).

Step 2: Generating hypotheses and formulating obstacles

The example in Box 8.1 exemplifies how a therapist might gather information
about clinically relevant factors, in a way that is guided by empirical research.
Once a therapist has gathered some clues about potential difficulties, the next
step involves the formulation of a hypothesis that explains how these factors
interfere with progress. In order to form hypotheses, it can be helpful to consider the following questions:

- What are the factors that seem relevant in this case?
- How might these factors make it difficult to cope with daily stressors?
- How might each factor interfere with a patient's goals?
- How might each factor interfere with change mechanisms?
- How might these factors interact with each other?

Box 8.2 provides an example of how to generate hypotheses, based on Annie's
case. The last question in Box 8.2 guides the therapist to draw a distinction

between *relevant risk factors* and *change mechanisms*. Mechanisms are concepts drawn from psychological theory. For example, in Annie's case, hypothesized change mechanisms involve rumination about past events, social avoidance and biased expectations about interpersonal contact. Relevant factors are concepts drawn from the empirical literature on prognostic indicators, as listed in Figure 8.2. This second troubleshooting step requires the therapist to form a hypothesis about how specific *factors interfere with the expected action of change mechanisms*. This is how we understand why some patients respond well and others respond less well to therapy: under ordinary circumstances, the application of change mechanisms should lead to improvements, but in some cases the excepted effects of these mechanisms are blocked or undermined by specific factors. This formulation process should result in the development of an *idiographic formulation*: a person-specific theory that enables the therapist and patient to make sense of what needs to change and what might be interfering with change.

Box 8.2 Generating hypotheses in Annie's case

What are the factors that seem relevant in this case?
Risk factors: loneliness and isolation.

Process factors: homework non-adherence, negative thoughts and emotional/behavioural reactivity to those thoughts.

How might these factors make it difficult to cope with daily stressors?
Annie faces several stressors in a typical week:

- getting on with college assignments
- observing other young people's lives/accomplishments on social media and comparing herself to them
- receiving messages from others and trying to decide how to respond
- dealing with daily chores (eating, cleaning, washing) while feeling deeply depressed.

Spending a lot of time in isolation and with negative thoughts induces a state of exhaustion, low mood and hopelessness. Examples of negative thoughts include:

- 'I am not as interesting, pretty and successful as others'
- 'I'm useless'
- 'I'm a pathetic child and others will eventually find out and reject me'.

She then avoids therapy tasks (e.g., making contact with friends via social media) because she is too depressed and fearful about the consequences of reaching out to others, but also does not expect that this will be helpful to her.

How might each factor interfere with the patient's goals?
As a consequence of the above factors, she is not on track because she is not making progress towards her personal goals (socializing, getting a job, dating) and is avoiding doing the things that might enable her to feel better.

How might each factor interfere with change mechanisms?

Homework non-adherence: While Annie avoids making social contact, she will never be able to get used to being around people and she will not be able to disconfirm or modify her beliefs and expectations about interpersonal life (her fear of rejection will remain fixed).

Loneliness/isolation: A lack of company and/or activities outside of her room probably mean that she has very low stimulation and opportunities to gain a sense of pleasure or distraction. This lack of stimulation traps her in a situation where most of her energy is focused internally on her own thoughts. This contributes to a chronic pattern of rumination. Rumination is a process that maintains her low mood, which in turn makes it difficult to motivate herself to take steps towards fulfilling her goals.

It is good practice to generate such a hypothesis and formulation in consultation with a clinical supervisor or another experienced therapist. The reason for consultation is to enable us to sense-check our hypotheses, but also to change or refine our hypotheses with another therapist's input. This ensures that our hypothesis is not overly influenced by our own biases or intuitions. During clinical supervision, you can work through the above questions alongside a supervisor to generate possible hypotheses and to arrive at the most plausible formulation based on information gathered through the initial discussion with the patient.

We had a question on our end-of-session questionnaire that was formulated as 'The therapist tells me what he thinks about me'. One of my patients suddenly started to fill out 'not really', whereas in all the previous sessions they had filled it out with 'not at all'. So, in the session, I showed the results to the patient and I asked him what was going on. And then he said, 'Well, you know what, you are really nice and very supportive because you are a psychologist, but, in reality, you think completely differently about me. You think I am a loser, and that I should have finished my studies a long time ago.' Having the feedback made me really aware that there was mistrust, that I otherwise would have missed completely. Because of it, I was able to talk with the patient about it and to repair the therapeutic relationship.
                    – Wolfgang Lutz, feedback researcher and CBT therapist

Step 3: Developing a troubleshooting plan

Once you have generated a plausible hypothesis and formulation, the next step is to generate an action plan in consultation with a peer or supervisor. To achieve this, it can be helpful to consider the following questions:

- Which of these factors could be amenable to therapeutic change? How?
- Which of these factors are less amenable to therapeutic change?

- Which *supportive* factors might mitigate the influence of *complicating* factors?
- Who else could help to increase support or resources?

Some clinically relevant factors can be directly targeted and modified through therapy, such as low expectancy or alliance ruptures. However, some factors cannot be changed at all (e.g., life events such as bereavement), or at least not through psychotherapeutic strategies (e.g., financial difficulties). The first two questions prime us to consider whether we should directly attempt to *modify* clinically relevant factors (e.g., alliance), whether we need to work *with* these factors (e.g., adjust therapy to the patient's cultural world-view), or whether we need to work *around* these factors (e.g., gaining the trust of a highly suspicious patient in order to promote collaboration with therapy tasks, not expecting that their suspiciousness towards all other people will fundamentally change). Coming back to Annie's case, the therapist needs to work with her age-related world-view and goals, work around her isolation in the short-term (not forcing her to socialize immediately), and attempt to modify her low expectancy about the effects of social exposure tasks, which may later 'modify' her isolation.

Step 4: Implementing the troubleshooting plan

Once an action plan has been generated based on a plausible hypothesis and formulation, the therapist should implement this plan as part of the therapy process. In keeping with the principle of *collaboration* outlined above, the therapist should always share their formulation openly with the patient to instil a sense of trust, transparency and teamwork. It is a good idea to convey such a formulation in lay terminology, avoiding technical jargon or overcomplicated language. This prepares a patient to consider the action plan that is logically related to the formulation. Following the principles of *personalization* and *experimentation* outlined above, therapist and patient should come to an agreement about which actions, changes or adjustments to the therapy plan will be tried out. Such a plan should be framed as an experiment based on a plausible hypothesis. We might expect to see specific changes after trying certain actions or adjustments to the plan. As in experimental psychology, we cannot be certain if such a plan will or will not work, but the best way to find out is to try it out and to observe what happens.

Step 5: Evaluating the troubleshooting plan

Following the principle of *empiricism* outlined above, our troubleshooting plan must be evaluated in the same way that we would approach a scientific experiment: using data in order to assess if expected changes occur or not. In feedback-informed treatment, we use ROM and feedback graphs to evaluate our troubleshooting plan. If symptoms are back on track after implementing our plan, then this gives us reasonable evidence that our plan worked. However, if symptoms are consistently NOT before, during and after we have implemented our plan, this gives us reasonable evidence that our plan did not work.

Step 6: Reviewing the overall treatment plan

The final step in this troubleshooting process involves making decisions about the treatment plan depending on the outcome of the prior step. A different course of action will be necessary depending on whether the implementation of the action plan led to an objectively improved trajectory of symptoms or not. If progress is back on track, there are two possible decisions that the therapist could consider: resuming standard evidence-based treatment or offering an adapted form of treatment based on the troubleshooting plan. The first option is appropriate in cases where a modifiable factor has been successfully dealt with, and which no longer complicates the course of treatment. An example of this scenario would be a case where an alliance rupture has been successfully repaired, and therefore the standard course of treatment can continue unhampered by alliance problems. The second option is appropriate in cases where therapy needs to be personalized or adapted to work with or work around a factor that is not feasible to modify. For example, it is appropriate for the therapist to continually adapt the treatment style or plan to fit a patient's cultural world-view or personality traits, both of which are clinically relevant factors that are not easily modifiable. Following the principles of *empiricism* and *collaboration*, decisions about the treatment plan should be made through consultation with the patient and a clinical supervisor.

If progress continues to be NOT despite the therapist's best efforts to implement the action plan, this opens up two possibilities. First of all, a persistent NOT trajectory should be taken as evidence that the action plan did not work. It may be because the hypothesis, formulation and/or action plan were inadequate. Therefore, one possible response is to go back to Step 2 outlined above and to restart the process of clinical troubleshooting, again in consultation with a clinical supervisor and the patient. A second possible course of action is to consider an augmented or different form of treatment. This second course of action implies that the current treatment is insufficient or inappropriate to meet the patient's needs. This might result in the augmentation of the current therapy with other forms of support (e.g., pharmacotherapy, financial or social support) or a conclusion of the treatment plan and referral to another treatment (e.g., a different type of treatment or service).

Decisions about ending a treatment and/or recommending another form of treatment should be sense-checked with a clinical supervisor, due to its potential consequences on the patient's wellbeing. Such decisions may also be constrained by the service context and policies. For example, therapists working in short-term therapy services may only have sufficient time to implement a troubleshooting plan for a finite number of sessions before they are obliged to consider other treatment options. However, therapists working in private practice or in services that allow long-term therapy may have more flexibility to restart the troubleshooting cycle and to continually adapt therapy to best fit the patient's characteristics and needs.

Conclusions

All therapists will encounter moments in their clinical practice where treatment is not progressing well. After determining if a lack of progress or a certain amount of worsening of symptoms or functioning is evident, the question arises: 'What do we do now?' In this chapter we have discussed clinical trouble-shooting methods that can help therapists to assess relevant factors that might get in the way of progress, and to decide whether an adaptation in the treatment is needed in a structured way. We emphasize the idiographic (person-specific) nature of clinical obstacles and solutions and the usefulness of adopting a scientist–practitioner mindset when dealing with such obstacles.

Key points in this chapter

- Clinical troubleshooting is a process that brings the scientific method into psychotherapy practice. It requires the therapist to observe and measure progress objectively, using routine outcome monitoring as a key source of information.
- If therapy is not on track, the therapist explores relevant factors, forms a plausible hypothesis, develops an action plan, tests this plan empirically, and comes to a reasoned decision based on the evidence.
- We consider that this process, summarized in Figure 8.1, brings science and practice together for the benefit of patients.

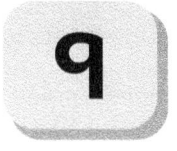

Integrating outcome monitoring and feedback in clinical supervision

In this chapter

Previous chapters discussed how to select, administer and integrate outcome measures and progress feedback into psychological therapy practice. This chapter provides a guide on how to integrate ROM and feedback into the wider context of clinical supervision and clinical case discussions in healthcare teams. The chapter begins by providing a brief review of relevant literature in the field of clinical supervision. This covers key theories on the functions of clinical supervision, its related tasks and the empirical literature investigating the impact of supervision and supervisory training. Research findings related to the limitations of traditional supervision methods serve as a basis to propose a clinical outcome oriented supervision model (COSMo) which is elaborated in the latter part of this chapter, along with practical suggestions on how to implement and evaluate such a model in managed healthcare organizations.

Clinical supervision theory

Supervision as a mechanism for ethical practice

Clinical supervision is a core aspect of ethical practice in psychological care and it is a feature of a therapist's career irrespective of their stage of professional development or level of competence. Indeed, many professional organizations require therapists to access supervision regularly as a requisite for ongoing accreditation. This requirement is enshrined in codes of conduct such as those published by the American Psychological Association, the British Psychological Association, the Dutch Association of Psychologists and other professional societies around the world that oversee the practice of psychological therapists. Common to these regulations and codes of conduct is the establishment of clinical supervision as a central mechanism to ensure that therapists practise in an ethical and effective manner, consistent with principles outlined in the

Universal Declaration of Ethical Principles for Psychologists (International Union of Psychological Science, 2008). Such principles require therapists to practise in a way that demonstrates: (1) respect for the dignity of people; (2) competent caring for their well-being; (3) honesty and integrity; (4) professional and scientific responsibility. As such, clinical supervision should be structured in a way that these principles can be evidenced and adhered to. Various models of supervision have evolved over time to support ethical and effective practice in psychological therapy.

Theoretical models

The practice of psychological therapy is influenced by several theoretical orientations and perspectives about mental health. Similarly, various theoretical models that define clinical supervision and specify its key functions have been documented in several books (e.g., Bernard & Goodyear, 2014; Driver & Martin, 2002; Fleming & Steen, 2004; Scaife, 2008; Stoltenberg & Delworth, 1987; Watkins & Milne, 2014). Some of these perspectives are grounded in and influenced by specific theoretical orientations such as psychodynamic therapy (e.g., Ladany et al., 2005), cognitive behavioural therapy (e.g., Liese & Beck, 1997), humanistic-existential therapy (Farber, 2010), group psychotherapy (Proctor, 2000), systemic therapy (Vetere & Sheehan, 2017) and others. Some theorists have taken a broader perspective, seeking to outline general principles and tasks that are essential to the ethical and effective supervision of psychotherapists from various orientations. Some influential historical developments are summarized in Box 9.1, although a comprehensive explanation of each is beyond the scope of this chapter.

Box 9.1 Different supervision models

Supervisory working alliance model
Building on his influential concept of the working alliance, Bordin (1983) conceptualized the supervisory working alliance as characterized by an affective bond and a formal agreement between the therapist and supervisor on specific goals and tasks. He proposed eight key goals: mastering therapy skills; understanding patients; awareness of process issues; awareness of self and impact on process; overcoming obstacles to learning and mastery; understanding concepts and theory; stimulating research; and maintaining service standards. He proposed that these goals could be met through a series of structured tasks: (1) the therapist prepares a report related to their practice and obtains feedback from the supervisor; (2) the supervisor observes the therapist's practice (i.e., *in vivo*, via recordings or transcripts) and offers feedback; (3) specific problems and issues are selected and prioritized for discussion in supervision, with connection to one or more of the above goals. As part of this process, the bond between the supervisor and therapist may be

experienced at different times in the form of a teacher–trainee, therapist–patient relationship.

Seven-eyed model

The process or 'seven-eyed' model of supervision (Hawkins & Shohet, 1989) proposes that the focus of supervisory discussions can focus on one of seven targets: (1) therapy session content; (2) therapeutic strategies; (3) patient-therapist relationship; (4) the therapist's internal experience; (5) the here-and-now process between supervisor and supervisee; (6) the internal experience of the supervisor; (7) the wider context.

Tripartite model

The tripartite model of supervision (Inskipp & Proctor, 2001) proposes that clinical supervision has three broad functions: a *normative* function that serves the purpose of quality assurance and ethical practice; a *formative* function that focuses on the development of skills and knowledge; and a *supportive* function that enables the therapist to resolve difficulties and to cope with the challenges inherent to therapeutic work.

Cyclical model

The cyclical model (Page & Wosket, 2001) proposes that supervision follows five phases in a recurring cycle: *contracting* establishes a mutual understanding about the supervisory goals, tasks, boundaries, roles and expectations; the supervisor and therapist *focus* on specific issues, objectives and priorities; a reflective *space* is established, promoting investigation, challenge, containment and affirmation; a *bridge* serves the function of consolidation and integration of learning and development across supervision meetings, and to set goals and plan actions; and a *review* stage serves the purpose of evaluating the supervisee's practice and how supervision is working, which can lead back to the start of the cycle.

Integrative–developmental model

The integrative-developmental model of supervision (Stoltenberg et al., 2014) proposes that psychotherapists develop over time through three distinctive levels: *novice*, *intermediate* and *advanced*. These levels of competence can be assessed across three broad domains of motivation to learn and develop: autonomy versus dependence on the supervisor; self-other awareness and sensitivity to interpersonal processes. The supervisory process is meant to be adapted to the particular level of competence displayed by the therapist across these domains. For instance, supervision for novice therapists may be more didactic, focusing on skill acquisition; supervision for intermediate therapists may focus on the development of a broader repertoire of therapy skills; and supervision for advanced therapists tends to be steered by the therapist, with an emphasis on integration across the three domains and mastery of therapy skills and techniques across a broad range of patients.

Supporting the development of the therapist's treatment competences (i.e., knowledge, attitudes, and skills) is a function that can be found across various supervisory models described in Box 9.1. There is ample evidence that interpersonal skills such as empathy are associated with positive treatment outcomes (e.g., see Anderson et al., 2016; Elliott et al., 2018). There is also replicated evidence that clinical outcomes are associated with the skilled delivery of evidence-based interventions (i.e., treatment integrity) measured by the combination of adherence and competence scores using structured evaluations by independent raters (Power et al., 2022). Consistent with this evidence, competency-focused approaches to clinical supervision have been proposed by several authors (e.g., Falender & Shafranske, 2004; Kaslow, 2004; Young et al., 2013). An extension to this approach is the proposal of specific competences for supervisors, such as the ability to apply educational principles, to enable ethical practice, to provide feedback, to foster culturally competent practice and to use outcome measures to assess progress (Roth & Pilling, 2008). In addition, theorists have proposed that clinical supervision should help to foster awareness of how diversity-related issues may impact the patient and therapy process and to promote culturally adapted and diverse-sensitive practice (Beck, 2016; Falender et al., 2013; Tsui et al., 2014). Related to this topic is the recognition of power imbalances in the patient-therapist and therapist-supervisor relationships (Patel, 2013; Tsui et al., 2014), which may at times influence the bond and relational process.

In spite of the diversity of theoretical models, there are nevertheless common definitions and functions that can be gleaned across the literature. Common to all models is the idea that clinical supervision is a relational process that involves an alliance between professionals (supervisee–supervisor; supervisee–peer group), with specific goals and related tasks.

Definition and functions

Broadly speaking, clinical supervision is a formal working alliance between a therapist and a supervisor or peer group, intended to fulfill three aims. First, it aims to guarantee the welfare of patients by ensuring ethical practice and decision-making. Second, it aims to foster effective practice in individual cases and over the course of a clinician's development. Third, it offers a supportive and reflective space to enable clinicians to solve problems and to cope with the emotionally demanding nature of therapy. These functions are inclusive of the ideas conveyed across various theoretical models, and are elegantly summarised in Inskipp and Proctor's (2001) tripartite model of supervision summarised in Table 9.1.

Goals, tasks and methods

Guided by the diverse models of supervision that have emerged in the field, there is a large array of goals with corresponding tasks and methods that are routinely employed in the supervision of psychotherapists. For example, the goal of developing skills in a specific therapeutic technique could be approached

Table 9.1 A clinical outcome-oriented interpretation of the tripartite model of supervision

Functions of supervision	Description and relation to outcome monitoring and feedback
Normative	Supervision as a quality assurance process, ensuring that therapy and clinical decision-making are conducted in an ethical manner, observing organizational expectations and professional codes of conduct.
	Adherence to evidence-based practice and routine outcome monitoring are related to this function.
Formative	Supervision as a practice-development process, enabling the clinician to acquire, practice, refine and master psychological theories, concepts and intervention strategies over time. This involves the identification of areas for development and deliberate practice of specific skills.
	The use of quantitative (i.e., measures) and qualitative (i.e., information elicited from patients, peers and supervisors) feedback is related to this function.
Supportive/ Restorative	Supervision as a reflective process, facilitating the resolution of clinical dilemmas and problems and the clinician's personal growth and adjustment to the challenges inherent to psychotherapeutic work.
	A collaborative focus on clinical trouble-shooting, aiming to identify and work around obstacles to effective therapy in cases that are not-on-track, is related to this function.

using various tasks (e.g., reading, observing, rehearsing, applying the skill with a patient, reflecting, obtaining feedback, etc.) and methods (live/audio/video observation, feedback from patient/supervisor, qualitative/quantitative feedback, etc.). Furthermore, as proposed by developmental models (e.g., Stoltenberg et al., 2014), the selection of goals, tasks and methods may depend on the supervisee's stage of professional development. A bewildering number and heterogeneous set of tasks are described in the literature concerning clinical supervision; such as case discussions, role plays, reflection on interpersonal processes, identification of practice development goals, observation of practice and corrective feedback, formal evaluation of practice using adherence/competence ratings, problem solving, coaching/mentoring on theory/practice, risk assessment, reflections about the role of power in relationships, considerations about diversity and cultural adaptation of therapy, reflection about the supervisory process itself, etc. For example, in one study investigating what supervisees did in clinical supervision, Milne and Gracie (2001) identified 20 discrete tasks, which raises the question: which tasks are actually necessary to support effective therapy?

A general reading of this literature gives the impression that 'anything goes' in clinical supervision. This situation has motivated some authors to take a critical stance and to attempt to define how an evidence-based model of supervision might be achieved (e.g., Milne, 2009) and which aspects of supervision might constitute good practice (e.g., Simpson-Southward et al., 2017). Accordingly, it is pertinent to ask how we can select supervisory goals, tasks and methods that might ultimately benefit therapists and patients. In the next section, we explore this question from the perspective of research in the field of psychological therapies.

Research on the impact of supervision and supervisory training

Over 50 narrative and systematic reviews of the empirical literature on clinical supervision have been published since the 1970s (e.g., Hansen & Warner, 1971; Tugendrajch et al., 2021). A common thread of discussion in these reviews is that, relative to the wider psychotherapy efficacy literature, the methodological quality of the research on clinical supervision is limited and characterized by high risk of bias (Ellis et al., 1996, 2008; Milne et al., 2012; Watkins et al., 2021). Although a methodological critique is beyond the scope of this chapter, common sources of bias includes problems with the reliability and validity of measures used, limited attention to patient outcomes, no tracking of change over time, no *a priori* hypothesis specification, small sample sizes, and selection and other sampling biases (i.e., lack of representative samples). As such, we are cautious about drawing strong conclusions from this literature. Nevertheless, it is possible to derive some lessons from these studies across a few themes described below.

Qualitative studies of supervisees' experiences often indicate that therapists generally perceive the supervisory relationship as central to its perceived benefits, which relate to their personal and professional development (Wheeler & Richards, 2007; Wilson et al., 2016). Supervision is perceived to enable therapists to increase self-awareness and to identify 'blind spots' in their practice. In particular, supervisees tend to see supervision as primarily serving an educational and evaluative function, which can often raise feelings of incompetence when the feedback they receive is discrepant to their expectations or wishes. These difficulties can be amplified in situations where there is a perceived power imbalance in the supervisee–supervisor relationship, or when the supervisor is perceived as punitive, unpredictable or unprofessional. Good supervisors are often perceived to have qualities such as consistency, empathy and warmth and are perceived to adjust their style according to the needs and preferences of the supervisee. In turn, studies that gather supervisors' views indicate that they perceived the most effective supervisees (based on their clinical outcomes) to be proactive, well prepared and organized for their supervision meetings, compared to other supervisees (Green et al., 2014). Supervisees perceive good supervision to lead to specific outcomes including increasing confidence and self-efficacy in therapy practice, increased self-awareness, increased awareness of relational dynamics/processes, improved ability to monitor and evaluate their work, ability to practise ethical decision-making, improved professional identity and job satisfaction, improved ability to manage challenges, higher motivation to approach difficulties in practice, improvements in therapeutic alliance and patient outcomes. Although the list of perceived benefits is impressive, the methodological limitations of qualitative studies preclude drawing strong conclusions about cause–effect relations. It is not possible to know if the respondents in these studies may have attained such benefits over time anyway, with the accumulation of clinical experience and irrespective of the supervisory quality or methods.

In contrast, reviews of quantitative studies draw more cautious conclusions. Broad-scope reviews of studies on the impact of supervision in psychological therapy (e.g., Freitas, 2002; Holloway & Neufeldt, 1995; Kühne et al., 2019; Ellis et al., 1996; Reiser & Milne, 2014; Watkins, 2011, 2020; Wheeler & Richards, 2007) and narrower reviews of supervision in specific therapies such as CBT (e.g., Milne & James, 2000; Alfonsson et al., 2018) typically report mixed and often inconclusive findings. More consistent support is found for the hypothesis that clinical supervision is generally acceptable to therapists, as indicated by typically high ratings of satisfaction and perceived helpfulness. Processes such as the therapeutic alliance and treatment competence appear to be associated with supervisory tasks. In particular, three experiential learning tasks appear to have greater empirical support for the development of therapist competence and self-efficacy: corrective feedback about practice/competence; educational role-play; and modelling (live/video demonstration) of therapy tasks (Milne et al., 2011). A recent review of the influence of different supervisory methods organized results according to formative (i.e., skill development) and restorative (i.e., organizational well-being) outcomes (Bradley & Becker, 2021). They concluded that formative outcomes were more convincingly associated with corrective feedback, intervention planning/discussion and role play, while restorative outcomes were associated with supervisory alliance and support (i.e., expressed via empathy and praise). Interestingly, other purportedly important aspects of supervision (e.g., caseload management discussions, tasks to enhance self–other process awareness, self-oriented reflection and practice of therapy skills, multicultural orientation, reflection on power relations, etc.) count with no convincing empirical support.

Importantly, a consistent conclusion across quantitative reviews is that patient outcomes are often neglected in clinical supervision research and the studies that do include patient outcomes offer weak and inconclusive evidence. Furthermore, the 'good supervisor' constructed through qualitative studies does not appear to exist in the real world. Replicated large-scale studies investigating supervisor effectiveness did not find evidence of variability in outcomes attributable to different supervisors (Rousmaniere et al., 2016; Whipple et al., 2020), and hence there is little empirical justification to conclude that there are more and less clinically effective supervisors. Moreover, the latter studies found no evidence of associations between patient treatment outcomes with supervisor experience, level of training or theoretical orientation. At most, we can say that some supervisors are better educators than others, particularly if they apply experiential learning tasks such as those described above. In conclusion, some supervision tasks can help therapists' skill development and occupational well-being, but a direct influence on patient outcomes is not evident.

COSMo: A clinical outcome-oriented supervision model

Making a case for outcome-oriented supervision

Clinical guidelines for the treatment of mental health problems stipulate that evidence-based psychological therapy should be delivered by qualified clinicians who practise under regular supervision (e.g., APA, 2015; NICE, 2011). Accordingly, professional psychological therapy organizations in several countries require therapists to access a minimum number of supervision hours in order to obtain and maintain their accreditation. In England, for example, therapists working in the national Improving Access to Psychological Therapies (IAPT) programme are required to access the equivalent of one hour of clinical supervision per full-time working week (National Collaborating Centre for Mental Health, 2018). In other settings, supervision is accessed on a less frequent basis, but most therapists engage in supervision at several points during their career, in particular during initial training and while training to deliver new interventions. Therapists spend a considerable amount of time accessing and delivering supervision throughout their career. To a great extent, supervision is uncritically accepted as a valuable and essential aspect of practice by educators, trainees, therapists and supervisors. This view is reified in clinical guidelines, training curricula and highly cited textbooks in the field.

A close reading of the scientific literature on clinical supervision in psychological therapy raises serious questions about its merits. Therapists can spend time in supervision carrying out a wide array of tasks that may or may not be of clinical or professional value. Yet, it seems that the majority of supervisees tend to provide high satisfaction ratings. However, it is entirely possible to be satisfied with a comfortable form of supervision that is characterized by empathy and praise, but which may be clinically inert if it does not challenge the therapist to stretch beyond their comfort zone, to learn and to develop further. Previous authors have also described accounts and evidence that supervision can sometimes drift into 'collusion' (Milne et al., 2009) or 'game playing' (McIntosh et al., 2006). *Collusion* can take the form of a collegial relationship where the supervisee is not challenged in any significant way and whatever they say or do is positively reinforced by the supervisor. *Game playing* can take the form of power games (e.g., discussions intended to assert authority and expertise) or by acting out dysfunctional interpersonal patterns (e.g., coercion, bullying). Alas, it is not surprising that research in the field has found little or no effects of clinical supervision on patient-level clinical outcomes.

Ultimately, we agree with other authors that improving outcomes for patients is the 'acid test' for clinical supervision (Ellis & Ladany, 1997) and this should be the primary goal and metric to assess its value. Other – associated – goals such as trainee development and well-being (i.e., formative and supportive/restorative aspects) are secondary and in the service of the primary goal of offering safe and effective treatment. In this supervision model, we do not focus on therapists' personal growth or solely focus on theoretical and technical development, since we believe that other methods are better suited for that (e.g., personal therapy, clinical training). Ethical practice is effective and safe practice and, as such, clinical supervision should be primarily focused on improving clinical outcomes. Safety and effectiveness should be measured and monitored using psychometric tools, and we should be committed to improving outcomes by applying evidence-based methods. We propose that, in order for supervision to be a vehicle for the improvement of clinical outcomes, it is important to optimize supervision time by focusing on a circumscribed set of goals and tasks that have the best probability of influencing clinical outcomes.

Aims and structure of a clinical outcome-oriented supervision model

COSMo has three broad aims:

- *Amplify* what works: Developing and refining interpersonal skills, treatment adherence and competence (i.e., treatment integrity).
- *Rectify* what is not working: Using progress feedback and clinical troubleshooting strategies for cases that are not-on-track.
- *Support* and restore: Enabling professional development, ethical practice and preventing burnout.

To fulfill these aims, COSMo is guided by a set of functions that have corresponding goals and tasks. Furthermore, clinical supervisors should develop and maintain specific competences to guide and support their supervisees effectively. This overall structure and competence framework is presented in Table 9.2. It is recommended that therapists and supervisors establish a formal written contract at the beginning of the supervisory relationship and also set a specific timeframe for the review of this contract and process. The supervisory contract should cover the following domains:

- Practical details, such as the frequency, duration and format (i.e., individual, group, in-person or online, etc.) of the supervision meetings.
- A list of specific goals-tasks-methods selected from the framework in Table 9.2, with an agreement on which will be prioritized during a specific timeframe.

- An explicit and detailed agreement on a routine outcome monitoring strategy that will enable the therapist to monitor their outcomes, to obtain patient-reported feedback, and to support the development of their practice development plan.
- An agreement on how difficulties and potential disagreements will be raised and addressed in a professional way.
- An agreement on how often the supervisory process will be formally reviewed, allowing regular opportunities for feedback between supervisor and supervisee or group members in a group supervision context.

Considerations about the agenda of meetings, the style of supervision and the relational bond

COSMo supervision meetings are guided by a specific set of goals and competencies outlined in Table 9.2, all in the service of improving patients' treatment outcomes. In order to focus maximum attention on the tasks that are most likely to improve clinical outcomes, supervision meetings should be structured by an agenda. As a minimum, the agenda of each meeting should cover the following areas:

- A review of the current status (i.e. are they on track or not on track?) of patients' treatment outcomes [goal F1]
- A focused review of cases that are not on track, as a priority for the meeting, and following the methods outlined in Table 9.2 [goal S1]
- Reviewing or developing a risk management plan for any patients where there are concerns about their safety or the safety of others [goal N2].

Other domains, goals and tasks can be included depending on time availability, and after covering the three areas listed above, which are deemed to be a priority and most likely to support clinical improvements and to prevent adverse incidents.

COSMo is intended to support therapists to integrate feedback as part of their clinical practice and professional development. As such, measurement is central to most of the competences listed in Table 9.2. Feedback from patients is regularly obtained via ROM and feedback, as well as qualitative accounts from therapy sessions. Feedback from supervisors is used to support the therapist's practice development and to refine and improve their skills over time. Feedback from supervisors is obtained in two ways: (1) via formal observations and ratings of adherence and/or competence in the delivery of evidence-based therapy; and (2) via observation of specific therapy skills rehearsed via role playing exercises within the supervisory meetings. We recommend that the specific rating tools for the first type of feedback (adherence/competence) are consistent with the therapist's clinical qualifications and theoretical orientation. Aspects of the therapist's practice should be observed by supervisors frequently (e.g., at least every 3–4 supervision sessions), either via recordings of actual therapy

Table 9.2 COSMo: functions, goals, tasks, methods and competences

Function	Goals	Tasks	Methods	Supervisor competences
Normative	Deliver therapy with integrity [N1]	• Observe clinical practice • Rate clinical practice • Provide feedback on adherence and competence	• Observation of clinical practice (*in vivo*, audio, video) • Use formal adherence/competence rating scale matched to the evidence-based therapy model/protocol	• Familiarity with the treatment model/protocol • Ability to provide quantitative and qualitative feedback on observed practice • Ability to deliver corrective feedback on skills deficits and specific instruction on deliberate practice tasks
	Evaluate and manage risk [N2]	Discuss/agree a risk management plan.	• Review quantitative outcome measures • Focus on any specific indicators of risk • Consider other qualitative sources of information • Consider risk and protective factors • Formulate a plan of action	• Ability to select and interpret outcome measures that capture data on risk factors such as self-harm, suicide and interpersonal threats • Familiarity with theoretical models for suicidal risk and relevant empirical evidence
	Practice in line with professional, ethical and organizational standards [N3]	Identify and address malpractice	• Observation of clinical practice (live, audio, video) • Discuss other evidence, such as reports of 'near miss' incidents, adverse incidents or complaints • Identification of specific aspects of poor practice and provision of corrective feedback (in line with expected standards) • Formulation of an action plan to improve practice • Use a learning model to aid discussion (e.g., Kolb's learning cycle model)	• Ability to guide supervisees towards ethical and professional practice, in a way that is sensitive and supportive • Ability and commitment to take appropriate corrective actions, in line with organizational policies, to protect patients from malpractice

(continued)

Table 9.2 (Continued)

Function	Goals	Tasks	Methods	Supervisor competences
Formative	Gain insight into therapeutic effectiveness [F1]	Evaluate: • outcomes for individual patients • aggregated outcomes at a caseload level • overall effectiveness relative to clinical norms	• Reliable change index using ROM • Reliable change and pre-post treatment effect sizes using ROM • Compare % reliable change and effect sizes to clinical benchmarks • Determine if patients are currently on track or not on track (Chapter 7)	• Interpretation of ROM • Awareness of and ability to interpret relevant clinical benchmarks
	Gain insight into therapeutic challenges [F2]	• Present a clinical case • Reflect on characteristics of the case that raise potential challenges • Form a hypothesis about how/why these challenges arise and how they could be addressed	• Written/oral presentation (assessment, formulation, treatment plan, process, outcomes) • Structured reflection guided by Figure 8.2 • Formulation of a hypothesis using the hypothesis-generating questions in Step 2 of the clinical trouble-shooting method (Chapter 8)	• Awareness of empirical literature on: o predictors of treatment outcomes o evidence-based change processes o cultural competence and adaptation of therapy • Ability to guide the therapist to apply clinical trouble-shooting methods

Table 9.2 (*Continued*)

Function	Goals	Tasks	Methods	Supervisor competences
	Formulate and implement a professional development plan [F3]	• Identify specific areas for practice development • Set specific goals • Set an action plan with a specific timeline for evaluation • Evaluate progress against goals	• Give priority to areas of development that are identified by and related to the goals/tasks listed above [N1-N3, F1-F2] • SMART development goals (specific – measurable – achievable – relevant to the above goals – and time-bound) • Deficits related to effective use of ROM and feedback should also be prioritised (Chapter 6) • Evaluate progress using ROM, goal-specific scales and supervisor ratings of observed practice	• Ability to guide development tasks using learning models, measures of treatment adherence/competence and benchmarking methods for ROM
Supportive	Improve outcomes for patients who are not on track [S1]	• Identify and address challenges to effective therapy for specific patients, in a personalized way	• Use ROM and feedback tools to identify NOT cases • Apply clinical trouble-shooting skills to adapt therapy for NOT cases	• Interpretation of ROM • Familiarity with the use of progress feedback methods/tools • Familiarity with the clinical trouble-shooting method

(continued)

Table 9.2. (Continued)

Function	Goals	Tasks	Methods	Supervisor competences

	Reflect on and clarify sources of difficulty in practice and occupational wellbeing [S2]	• Reflect on and clarify sources of difficulty in practice and well-being
		• Set goals to achieve in relation to occupational well-being
		• Set an action plan with a specific timeline for evaluation
		• Evaluate progress against goals
			• Supportive goals are different to those specified above [F3], and they should focus on the supervisee's wellbeing at work
			• Use a learning model to explore and reflect on potential sources of difficulty
			• Refer to the reward-imbalance and demands-resources models of burnout to foster awareness of job and organizational factors that may be relevant
				• Familiarity with literature on occupational burnout:
				  o job demands-resources model
				  o reward imbalance model
				  o job crafting model
				• Familiarity with learning models

sessions, or simulations via role play exercises (i.e., using the deliberate practice approach by Rousmaniere and Vaz using ultra-short targeted role play; see Boswell and Constantino, 2022 for CBT; and Goldman et al., 2021 for EFT). This will ensure that corrective feedback is regularly available, providing the best opportunity to support deliberate and frequent practice.

> *In supervision, our trainees usually bring a video clip from the session and the supervisor and trainee also have all the information from the ROM and clinical support tools, which offers several suggestions on what to do. So then, the supervisor and trainee talk about the case, what is going on, how valid the suggestions from the feedback system are and which ones might fit best for the next step in the treatment. That way you always consider the complete situation, because in the end it is still a clinical decision. Just a more data-informed decision, based on the information that the feedback system provides.*
> – Wolfgang Lutz, feedback researcher and therapist, Germany

In terms of its philosophy and style, this supervision model acknowledges the limits of clinical experience and judgement, and breaks away from the tradition of 'expert clinicians' mentoring others to develop expertise. There is little evidence to support the idea that a growth in years of clinical experience, qualifications or age lead to better psychological therapy outcomes (e.g., Wampold & Owen, 2021). Most therapists have blind spots, biases and limitations and no single therapist is able to help all of their patients to attain reliable and measurable improvements in their symptoms and functioning. This model assumes that all therapists have room for improvement and ongoing development in knowledge and skills. What matters most is the process of outcome-oriented supervision, feedback and commitment to ongoing development. The supervisor's level of qualifications or experience are less important by comparison to their ability to hold the structure of the supervisory process as described in this chapter. Insights about the causes and solutions of clinical dilemmas emerge from the process of clinical troubleshooting referred to in Table 9.2 (goal S1) and elaborated in Chapter 8 of this book. This supervision model can be seen as a process to foster a *growth mindset* in relation to psychological therapy practice – an attitude and belief that one's capacity to support people is continually a 'work in progress'. Acknowledging and discussing this philosophical stance is important from the very start, at the initial contracting meeting, and at regular review points.

Regarding the supervisory alliance, we follow Bordin's (1983) concept focusing on goals-tasks-bond, and have detailed the key goals and tasks that require agreement between supervisor and supervisees in Table 9.2. As for the bond, we expect that this may oscillate between feeling like a teacher–student relationship at times (i.e., for goals N1, N3, F3), or a patient–therapist relationship at other times (i.e., for goal S2). However, where possible, supervisors should continually monitor how the relational bond develops and they should openly discuss this with their supervisees, ideally aspiring to achieve a 'pilot–copilot' style of a supervisory bond. Ultimately, the therapist is the pilot in each of their clinical cases, and the supervisor's role is to support them to navigate this process and to become aware of their blind spots and difficulties.

In our supervision on progress feedback, we follow a coaching model and we try not to be the expert in the room, but rather a thought partner. I had a therapist come in once after the mother of the young person she was working with had signalled on a therapeutic alliance scale. The feedback showed that the mother was not feeling connected to the therapist. Initially, the therapist responded, 'Well, the mother did say that these questions were hard to understand, and I feel a really good relationship in the room, so maybe this does not mean much.' We started looking at the subscales and the items. It showed that the mother thought her child was not making enough progress. And so we zeroed in on that and I asked, 'What do you think progress means to this mom? What do you think she is expecting to see at this point in therapy?' And the therapist was able to say, 'I am not sure, but those are pretty good questions and I'll take them back to the next session.' So, the therapist was able to move away from her initial rejection of the feedback and move towards being curious about what was going on. In the next coaching session, the therapist told me that the mother had very high expectations and that through the feedback, they had been able to have a good conversation about what progress normally looks like.

    – Susan Douglas, feedback coach and implementation researcher, USA

Supervisory competences, training and development

Table 9.2 outlines specific competences that supervisors should aim to develop in order to deliver this model of supervision in a way that maximises the chance that it will have an impact on patients' outcomes and therapists' practice development. These competences are linked to all of the three functions of supervision (normative, formative, supportive) and their relevant taxonomy of goals-tasks-methods. This competence framework could inform the training of clinical supervisors, which – following the principles of outcome-oriented supervision – should be based on experiential tasks (i.e. role playing, recorded observation) and constant availability of corrective feedback from educators and/or peers. Having supervisors work according to this model will likely require additional training, in which the topics outlined in this chapter are covered, providing a portfolio of practice development materials and evidence of evaluation, followed by experiential training, for example being supervised on their own therapies according to this model for a period of time and getting feedback on supervising others according to this model.

    In some clinical settings, it has become common practice for clinical supervisors to access 'supervision of supervision' or 'meta-supervision' – for instance, through formal meta-supervision meetings with an experience clinical supervisor, scheduled at regular intervals. In our view, such an arrangement is inconsistent with the principles of the COSMo model. The meta-supervision approach assumes a hierarchy of competence, where there is an 'expert' supervisor that can mentor less expert supervisors, and which is inconsistent with the philosophy outlined above. Furthermore, there is no convincing evidence that meta-supervision influences clinical outcomes for patients. Instead, we propose that infrequent (i.e. quarterly, twice or once per year) supervisory practice development groups involving multiple supervisors could be a productive way to enable supervisors to share their experiences and to learn from each other. These events could be structured in such a way that participants can share examples of specific goal-task-method-outcome case examples linked to the competency framework outlined above. Furthermore, these events could involve participants in structured troubleshooting discussions about supervision-related challenges or dilemmas, using the same clinical troubleshooting framework described in this book (see Chapter 8).

Conclusions

Ethical guidelines in the field of psychological therapy require clinical practice to be effective and safe. Safety and effectiveness can and should be measured and monitored using psychometric tools. Measurement of clinical outcomes, observation of practice and corrective feedback should be central components of ethical and effective clinical supervision. Effective supervision involves focusing on the minimum necessary goals and tasks that have the best available evidence to refine clinical competences and to improve patients' outcomes. Improving clinical outcomes through supervision is hard to achieve and even harder to evidence. For these reasons, in this chapter we have made a case for a clinical outcome-oriented supervision model (COSMo) which integrates feedback as a central component among a small set of supervisory tasks that are most likely to make a positive difference to patients. This chapter provides a detailed taxonomy of functions, goals, tasks, methods and supervisory competences, as a practical guide for practising clinicians, supervisors and educators.

Key points in this chapter

- Studies show that routine clinical supervision meetings are typically quite heterogeneous, where a diverse array of tasks can be covered in a more or less structured way. Research evidence indicates that, of all these tasks, only a small set actually work to improve clinical competences: corrective feedback about practice/competence, educational role play and modelling (i.e. live or video demonstration).
- Research indicates that there is little evidence that clinical supervision influences patients' treatment outcomes, and this is likely to be due to the lack of consistent implementation of effective strategies listed above.
- COSMo is a model of clinical supervision that integrates measurement, feedback and effective supervisory tasks that have the best chance of making a positive impact on patients' health and functioning.

10 Consolidating practice and embracing future challenges

In this chapter

In this text, we have set out the principles and procedures for a transtheoretical, pragmatic, and practice-based approach to implementing ROM and clinical feedback informed treatment in routine clinical settings. In adopting a practice-based approach to ROM and feedback, we consider this to provide the greatest flexibility for practitioners to develop and integrate a ROM system that is consistent with their clinical practice. In this final chapter, we focus on aspects to consolidate ROM and feedback in the psychological therapies and then move to consider various challenges and potential developments for this field.

The previous chapters, having started by presenting the historical and scientific background to ROM (Chapter 1), took us through a natural sequencing of the associated methods and clinical skills and activities associated with ROM. These can be viewed as falling into three key phases. The first phase focuses on *preparing and collecting patient data* and comprises selecting the tools (Chapter 2); considering the barriers and enablers to implementing ROM (Chapter 3); addressing problems of adherence (Chapter 4); and introducing ROM to patients (Chapter 5). The second phase focuses on *therapist receipt of ROM data and feeding back data to patients* and comprises interpreting scores and patterns of data (Chapter 6) and recognizing when patients are not progressing as might be expected (Chapter 7). In response to such situations, the third phase focuses on *adapting treatment in response to ROM data* and comprises clinical troubleshooting (Chapter 8) and integrating ROM into supervision (Chapter 9). Having presented the various phases and components involved, a final task of the current chapter is to consolidate the practice of ROM and to ensure its sustainability.

What will be apparent is that ROM is not a single activity; it does not comprise a single method or skill occurring at a single point in time and involving only a single person. Rather, it is a complex activity that occurs over time, involving patients, therapists, data systems, and multiple levels of organizational involvement. But its purpose is simple: to improve the outcomes of patients, particularly of those who are not benefitting from treatment. Accordingly, in this chapter we provide a one-stop summary of the multiple steps involved.

A guideline to consolidating ROM and feedback-informed treatment

Here we summarize 15 key steps to help in the successful implementation of ROM and feedback-informed treatment.

Implementing ROM

These components are the precursors to applying ROM in clinical practice and are often the least considered. However, regardless of the views as to the impact of ROM, there is virtual unanimous agreement that the biggest issues that need to be addressed are those relating to implementation.

1 **Adopt the principle of ROM as a common standard of good practice:** ROM is an evidence-based component of therapy that, in most instances, provides an additive effect to treatment. It is not a panacea and will not yield additional gains with all patients, but it makes the outcomes of treatments transparent and gives patients a voice for communicating the impact of their presenting problems. To aid familiarity with ROM, we suggest:

- Reading accounts of the implementation of ROM and clinical feedback
- Becoming familiar with the research literature on ROM.

2 **Address organizational issues:** While it might appear that ROM is primarily a tool used by the therapist for a patient's benefit, it is important to appreciate that implementing ROM is an organizational intervention as it modifies clinical practice and involves being open about one's own work with patients. You will need to:

- Develop transparency about the rationale for the implementation of ROM
- Share information and involve other team members
- Set up meetings to air concerns and evaluate the potential impact
- Ensure all staff are onboard
- Address the hopes and fears of engaging in the various ROM components.

3 **Secure organizational and team support (e.g., technical, administrative, financial):** Because ROM comprises components outside of a therapy session – for example, the administration of an outcome measure – it is likely that it will involve administrative personnel. Such resources need to be available and willing to support ROM. We suggest:

- Being realistic about the level of support required
- Matching the level of implementation to the level of available support
- Include support staff in creating a culture of feedback in the organization
- Setting up a clinical outcome-oriented supervision model (COSMo).

4 **Decide on a timeline to assess implementation or when to evaluate (i.e., pilot):** When introducing an organizational intervention, it is often best to start small in order to make it manageable, learn from the initial

experience and then adapt and modify for wider implementation. It is important to:

- Be clear about the timeline for assessing the feasibility of implementation
- Select a time (by months) or cohort (by number of patients) so implementation is contained
- Set it up as a pilot, a collaborative learning venture
- Provide regular feedback on the success of implementation (e.g., monthly percentages of patients in which ROM and feedback is used).

5 **Identify leader and champion/champions:** Because implementing ROM is an organizational intervention, it requires leadership (visionary and operational) and also a champion(s) on the ground who are committed to ROM and can act as a link between management and practitioners. We suggest:

- Ensuring there is a leader or identified staff member with overall responsibility
- Using the enthusiasm of existing staff (e.g., is there is existing expertise/experience?).

Collecting ROM data

These components relate to the first phase outlined in the summary of chapters and comprise those activities associated with the generation of patient data.

6 **Select outcome measures that are both psychometrically sound and practical:** Arguably, the heart of ROM is the outcome measure as the value of the data depends on both the psychometric properties of the outcome measure and whether it is viewed by therapists as being a clinically meaningful instrument. It is important to:

- Select a measure(s) that is in general use in the service/clinic by practitioners
- Shorter measures are likely to be less of a burden for all personnel involved
- If set up as a pilot, then measures can be subsequently changed if the process doesn't work well
- If there are two good candidate measures, test out both in parallel or in series
- Select public domain or measures under Creative Commons licence to address copyright issues.

7 **Get to know as much about the selected measure(s) as possible:** Given that patients are being asked to complete a given measure on multiple occasions, it is important to become as familiar as you can with the measure, including individual items and their sensitivity to change. Make time to:

- Obtain and read the main measure development or review article
- Set up a training session with colleagues on the selected measure(s)
- Share people's experiences and expertise about the selected measure(s).

8   **Decide on the frequency of administration (i.e., the interpretation of routine):** It is important to generate sufficient data to be able to see patterns in the data or for software to produce expected treatment curves. It is likely that the shorter the planned treatment is, the more frequent is the need for data (i.e., at each session). We suggest:

- Selecting a frequency in line with the patient population and likely treatment duration
- Considering planned use of data to help inform frequency of administration.

Feeding back ROM data to patients

9   **Be clear as to how the measures will be used and shared with patients:** The benefit of ROM is the information it yields to enhance clinical observations and provide additional information upon which to base clinical decisions. It is therefore important to have a clear plan as to how the data will be used. We suggest:

- Considering and preparing for how ROM will integrate with individual clinical practice
- Sharing ideas and previous practice with colleagues
- Developing a personalized approach that is informed by the literature and experienced ROM users.

10   **Implement a system of clinical feedback using summary scores and simple graphs:** Using a feedback system that generates plots with expected treatment responses is most informative in stating when a patient's progress is deteriorating or not progressing in line with what might be expected from patients presenting with similar issues. If such software is not available, data can yield clear patterns that identify the need for reviewing the focus of therapy or identifying obstacles to progress. We suggest:

- Ensuring the ability to provide clinical feedback using summary scores, ideally with graphs
- Practise providing feedback with a willing colleague (role plays).

11   **Use individual changes in item scores to inform therapy sessions:** While total scores are often used to graph progress, they mask information at the level of individual items which might show subtle changes that provide a granular level of feedback. We suggest:

- Considering using individual items from questionnaires to inform the focus and content of sessions
- Observing and comparing the pattern of item responses across questionnaires over time.

Adapting treatment in response to ROM

These components capture the ultimate aim of ROM, namely to adjust treatment in light of the data that will then lead to bringing a patient's progress back on track and also reduce dropout from treatment. Importantly, while data can be derived from computer software, observations from graphical data combined with curiosity and insights from research can lead to the practice of clinical troubleshooting, which can result in adapting treatment plans.

12 **Use clinical support tools to help identify obstacles to progress in treatment:** Research evidence clearly shows that using clinical support tools yields better outcomes in helping therapists to identify obstacles to patient improvement. We recommend:

- Adopting specific measures that yield additional information in identifying obstacles to getting a patient back on track (e.g., Assessment for Signal Clients)
- Adopting these measures is especially important in more complex patients.

13 **Adopt clinical troubleshooting:** Clinical troubleshooting is informed by a therapist's knowledge of the empirical literature relating to three domains associated with a patient's response to treatment: contextual, process, and patient factors. These three domains provide areas for a therapist to explore and consider clinically relevant factors that may be impinging on a patient's progress and provide clues as to possible adaptations. We suggest:

- Generating hypotheses as to what obstacles are impeding progress
- Developing an idiographic formulation that addresses the obstacle together with a clinical supervisor
- Developing and implementing a therapeutic plan
- Evaluating through observation of the ROM data.

14 **Integrate ROM into clinical practice and supervision:** With practice and experience, the aim is to integrate ROM and all its components into regular clinical practice and supervision. We suggest:

- Practice, practice, and practice
- Being minded of Pablo Casals' attributed response when asked why, at 90, he still continued to practise upwards of 4–5 hours a day, 'Because I think I am making progress.'

Sustaining ROM

15 **Assess the use of ROM and feedback with each completed case and use this information to inform the development of your clinical practice and supervision:** As with all clinical skills, being open to self-reflection and feedback from your own data will provide opportunities for learning.

- In the beginning, use each case as a learning experience
- Note what works well and what does not work well
- Share experiences with colleagues in supervision
- Move towards integrating ROM in your routine clinical practice and supervision
- Create a culture of feedback that is present in all the organizational levels of your practice.

These 15 steps provide a possible template for practitioners implementing or wishing to enhance the development of ROM in their everyday practice. In effect, they focus on what might be viewed as the infrastructure for adopting and implementing ROM. However, much of the content in previous chapters has focused on the person-to-person interactions with patients and additional processes and procedures are required, which we address next.

Maintaining ROM skills: The role of supervision and deliberate practice

A simple premise for developing and maintaining in-session implementation skills for ROM is to view it as a clinical skill akin to other aspects of clinical work. The practice of ROM is best subsumed within standard procedures providing oversight of clinical practice, of which there are two key components: supervision and deliberate practice.

Supervision

As outlined in Chapter 9, ROM should be a central component of clinical supervision meetings, to support both the treatment of individual patients and the broader practice development of the therapist. Of course, how each practitioner uses ROM will differ, but the purpose of including it in supervision is to ensure that it informs clinical practice and learning.

Deliberate practice: a meta-level of clinical feedback

In addition to supervision, a key component in developing and maintaining ROM skills is to engage in deliberate practice. Much has been written about deliberate practice but it is useful to set out four key elements from the original writings of Ericsson (Ericsson et al., 1993) as follows:

• Be motivated and ensure effort can be spent on practice
• Set the task to the level that is appropriate to your level of experience
• Establish a system of immediate and effective clinical feedback
• Repeat the specific task again and again.

Deliberate practice can manifest in many forms, but from the points above it can be seen that the aim is to select one specific aspect of ROM and focus on that one element, getting clinical feedback, and then cycling round again and again until it is felt that the specific task has improved.

Examples of deliberate practice might include focusing on the very specific way in which the measures and the completion of them by a patient is brought into the session. This can be achieved by recording the speech and then playing it back as a form of immediate clinical feedback to oneself. Of course, this can also be carried out in a small group with other practitioners feeding back on the tone, pacing, selection of words, etc. But the principle of deliberate practice is to focus on a discrete part of the potential interaction and practise it intensely until it is felt that it comes across as intended. In this book, we have outlined a model of clinical supervision that focuses on improving the therapist's clinical outcomes as a primary goal (Chapter 9). We propose that the notion of deliberate practice is a central aspect of the *formative* function of clinical supervision, as summarized in Table 9.2.

Building a practice-based body of ROM evidence

With the infrastructure in place and the practice of ROM being implemented and maintained, focus can then turn towards building an evidence-base from ROM grounded in everyday practice. Recalling that graphing of ROM can yield a variety of shapes or patterns, practitioners will begin to see emerging clusters among the patients they see in therapy. As the data increases, patients can become grouped into these clusters and commonalities determined. Similarities will become apparent and practitioners will begin to develop a sense of the profiles of differing groups of patients, what has been referred to in the literature as *nearest neighbours*.

Future challenges and potential for ROM and clinical feedback

The activity of ROM and clinical feedback carries both challenges and potential. Here, we consider some challenges and then conclude with a view of the potential offered to practice by this activity. A recent review of research on ROM and feedback identified five aspects that require attention and which provide a focus for action (see McAleavey & Moltu, 2021).

First, it should not be assumed that all clinical contexts and populations are the same. There is an increasing recognition that both cultural context and diversity need to be recognized and taken into consideration. Hence, our call for fluidity and flexibility in the application of ROM and clinical feedback and the use of forward and backward translations when extending outcome measures to culturally diverse populations.

Second, there is a clear challenge for practitioners to have sufficient knowledge about how to make ROM work practically and use it in their clinical work. The data by itself will have no impact on patients unless practitioners provide the data with clinical meaning.

Third, the importance of the provision of a rationale and of collaboration with patients is crucial. If patients do not understand the reason or the purpose for the clinical feedback or feel it is a technique of the practitioner rather than a shared activity, then it is less likely to be effective.

Fourth, notwithstanding the agenda of shared activity, again the issue of context has a bearing and it may be that implementation needs to be adjusted at different phases in therapy, for example. This point reinforces our view that flexibility is a key principle of effective and responsive implementation.

And finally, there is a recognition that clinical training will be required to maximize the impact of ROM. In considering how best to encourage the adoption and implementation of ROM clinical feedback, the logical place to start is with the new generation of practitioners progressing through a variety of local, regional, and national training programmes in differing countries. The aim is to introduce aspiring practitioners to the potential advantages of working with ROM and integrating it into their developing practice. However, an important principle of any training programme is that it espouses flexibility in terms of the various components (i.e., measures) and procedures (i.e., frequency, etc.).

One component that largely defines the content derived from ROM is the specific outcome measure adopted by practitioners. Different services or clinics will likely adopt different measures in response to their own knowledge-base and experience. Moving forward, however, there will likely be new measures developed that are specifically focused on the purpose of providing clinical feedback. The vast majority of outcome measures currently being used were not designed specifically for the purposes of clinical feedback. One component is the measure length (i.e., number of items). There has been a gradual move towards shorter measures that has coincided with the rise of ROM and clinical feedback procedures. However, measures reflect social times and values and it is reasonable to expect that new measures will be developed and would be considered for adoption.

However, a challenge in future years will be to ensure that ROM systems adopt a multi-domain perspective rather than becoming frozen by being constrained to a single measure. The irony could be that as an increasing body of data becomes available, there is a reluctance to modify or adapt the measurement. If and when the focus moves to other areas such as quality of life, significant changes will be necessary at a national level.

Towards data-informed and personalized practice

While the previous chapters have focused on adopting and implementing ROM and feedback with minimal technical support beyond what is standardly available (e.g., spreadsheet, software) – that is, no or lo-tech – it is clear that the field is a fast developing one and that data-informed practice will inevitably underpin the future commissioning and delivery of the psychological therapies (Lutz, Schwartz et al., 2022). Currently, in terms of moving towards data-informed practice that utilizes ROM and feedback as a central and integrated component, widespread adoption of a standardized software package or app is likely to be more successful than highly sophisticated packages that are beyond the financial limits of routine services. While the latter provide the scientific advances that are necessary to further the field, the agenda to improve practice requires widespread adoption.

It is likely that there will be an increasing market for software that maps and plots routine outcome data in the future. Technical development and increasing levels of sophistication will likely result in more informative and clinically useful packages. For example, contemporary studies show a trend towards the development of feedback systems that include automated decision tools to predict outcomes, to predict dropout, and to decide which type of treatment strategy may be helpful for not-on-track cases (Lutz, Deisenhofer et al., 2022). Furthermore, hi-tech dynamic clinical prediction systems are now capable of predicting treatment outcomes with greater precision than rational methods or expected treatment response curves (e.g., Bone et al., 2021). Future ROM and feedback systems are certain to become more accurate (more reliable predictions of relevant outcomes), less burdensome (through online data collection mechanisms), and more clinically useful than before (including clinical support tools). We foresee that technological advances will continue to propel the field of ROM, measurement-based, and data-informed treatment forward in the future. Still, we consider that the principles of good practice and idiographic (person-specific) assessment and trouble-shooting outlined in this book offer a solid foundation upon which psychological therapists can engage with measurement technology and integrate it into their clinical work.

List of interviewees

Throughout the book, we have used quotes from interviews with several therapists and researchers. The interviews were conducted by Kim de Jong. Below, the full list of interviewees and their affiliations are provided.

Robbie Babins-Wagner, PhD., CEO, Calgary Counselling Centre; Sessional Instructor and Adjunct Assistant Professor of Social Work, University of Calgary, Canada.

Heidi Brattland, PhD, Postdoctoral Fellow and Clinical Psychologist at St. Olavs University Hospital, Trondheim, Norway.

Susan Douglas, PhD, Assistant Professor of the Practice, Vanderbilt University; Clinical Product and Innovation Lead, Mirah; Executive and Team Coach, Coaching Supervisor, and Psychologist, United States.

Hidde Kuiper, MA, licensed clinical psychologist, registered cognitive behavioural therapist, Dokter Bosman, Amsterdam; GGz Centraal, the Netherlands.

Wolfgang Lutz, PhD, Professor of Clinical Psychology and Psychotherapy, University of Trier, Germany.

John Mellor-Clark, MSc, Owner/Managing Director, CORE IMS Ltd, United Kingdom.

Scott D Miller, PhD, Founder of the International Center for Clinical Excellence and co-founder of the Institute for the Study of Therapeutic Change, United States.

Christian Moltu, PhD, Professor II of Health and Caring Science, Western Norway University of Applied Science; Chairman of the Board, Norse Feedback; Chief Advisor, District General Hospital of Forde, Norway.

Andrew Page, PhD, Professor of Psychology and Pro Vice-Chancellor (Research), University of Western Australia, Australia.

Erik van der Put, MA, licensed clinical psychologist, registered cognitive behavioural therapist, owner of private practice Coaching en cognitieve gedragstherapie (CCGT), Chair of the Regional Alliance of Private Practices, PsyAlite GGZ ua, the Netherlands.

Terje Tilden, PhD, Modum Bad, Norway.

Glossary

American Psychological Association (APA)	The primary US professional body for psychologists.
ASEBA Brief Problem Monitor	An 18-item self-report measure to assess a person's problems (Achenbach et al., 2011).
Assessment for Signal Cases (ASC)	A 40-item questionnaire that measures internal and external therapy factors that may be hindering patient progress.
Beck Depression Inventory (BDI-II)	The second version of the Beck Depression Inventory comprising a 21-item self-report outcome measure of depression. It is a proprietary measure.
Brief Symptom Inventory (BSI)	A 53-item short outcome form of the SCL-90 that purportedly assesses nine subscales covering a range of symptoms. It is a proprietary measure.
CelestHealth – Behavioral Health Measure-20 (BHM-20)	A 20-item outcome measure that assesses wellbeing, symptoms and life functioning. It is a proprietary measure. There is a licence fee for its use.
Champions	Individuals in a clinical service who advocate the use of ROM, usually because they have had positive experiences using it.
Clinical Outcome oriented Supervision Model (COSMo)	A model of supervision that aims to amplify what works in therapy, rectify what doesn't and support the development of the therapist.
Clinical support tools (CSTs)	A set of supplementary questionnaires and clinical strategies that are used to support patients who are not responding well to treatment. These strategies target common problems related to the therapeutic alliance, motivation to change, difficult life events and social support. The techniques are described in manuals to guide therapists. Other contemporary clinical support tools include video instructions and cover other domains such as emotion regulation and self-harm risk management.

Clinical troubleshooting	A structured, six-step process, in which a therapist identifies obstacles that are interfering with treatment progress and makes a plan to systematically overcome these obstacles following a hypothesis-testing approach.
Clinical Outcomes in Routine Evaluation-Outcome Measure (CORE-OM)	A 34-item measure of psychological distress that assesses four domains: wellbeing, problems, functioning and risk. It is under a Creative Commons Licence and is therefore free to use.
Clinical Outcomes in Routine Evaluation-10 (CORE-10)	A 10-item short measure drawn from the CORE-OM. Items capture the domains of problems, functioning and risk. It is under a Creative Commons Licence and is therefore free to use.
Counseling Center Assessment of Psychological Symptoms (CCAPS-62 & CCAPS-34)	A 62-item and 34-item measure of psychological distress that was designed specifically for students. There is an annual membership fee.
Creative Commons Licence	A licence that states the associated material (measure) is free to use and to copy providing no changes are made to the content or form.
Expected treatment response (ETR)	The expected treatment response (ETR) model is a statistical forecast of treatment progress based on a set of patient variables. It provides the therapist with a visual set of parameters to judge if the patient's symptoms are on track or not-on-track to improvement.
Feedback-informed treatment	One term given to a form of ROM whereby treatment is adjusted in light of data from outcome measures.
Global Assessment of Functioning (GAF)	A single visual scale for measuring the extent to which a person's problems affect their daily functioning on a scale from 0 to 100. It derives from Axis V of the Diagnostic and Statistical Manual (DSM) and is therefore presumed to be copyrighted but free to use.
Holy Grail fallacy	The erroneous belief that a psychometric measure should measure all relevant aspects of a patient's health and goals, or else it is not worth using. This expression alludes to the common tendency for therapists to eschew using currently available and 'imperfect' measures, until they either design or find the 'Holy Grail' measure.

Improving Access to Psychological Therapies (IAPT)	A large, government-funded programme in England that provides a stepped-care approach to psychological therapies based on providing the least intensive intervention initially so as to make access easier. Patients who do not respond well to the initial step have the option to access more intensive psychological interventions. Patients with some conditions (e.g., post-traumatic stress disorder) are directly assigned to more intensive therapy.
Influencers	Role models who can have a positive impact in supporting ROM.
Measurement-based care	A term that is synonymous to ROM.
National Institute for Health and Care Excellence (NICE)	The influential UK body that produces clinical guidelines and standards across the whole range of mental and physical care.
Not-on-track (NOT) cases	Refers to patients whose current rate of improvement is not in line with what would be predicted based on patients presenting with similar conditions.
Omniscience fallacy	The erroneous belief that clinical judgement is the most trustworthy source of information regarding a patient's condition.
OQ System	A ROM system that uses the OQ-45 and developed by Michael Lambert and Gary Burlingame.
Ostrich syndrome	A process of being selective in only assimilating the positive from outcome measurement and not taking on board information that challenges a therapist's views.
Outcome Questionnaire (OQ-45.2)	The second revision of the OQW-45 comprising a 45-item measure of psychological distress tapping the domains of symptom distress, interpersonal relations, and social role (Lambert et al., 2004).
Outcome Rating Scale (ORS)	A 4-item visual analogue measure of the outcome of psychotherapy (Miller et al., 2003). It measures individual, interpersonal, social, and overall wellbeing). It is free to copy and use.
Partners for Change Outcome Management System (PCOMS)	A ROM system comprising the Outcome Rating Scale and the Session Rating Scale (Duncan & Reese, 2015).

Patient-focused research	A research approach, originated by Kenneth I Howard and his team, that focuses on deriving research insights from clinical data collected in routine care. The central focus is on understanding how individuals change during therapy, as opposed to the group-level perspective that is typical of clinical trials.
Patient Health Questionnaire-9 (PHQ-9)	A 9-item measure of depression, based on the criteria in the Diagnostic and Statistical Manual (DSM).
Practice-based evidence	A paradigm of research that places primary emphasis on routinely collected data as opposed to evidence drawn from clinical trials.
Progress monitoring	A term that is synonymous to ROM.
Randomized controlled trials	A research design in which patients are randomly assigned to one of two conditions, such as an intervention and a control group, while all other variables are held to be equivalent (e.g., balanced between groups).
Real-time monitoring	A term that is synonymous to ROM., but which emphasizes paying attention to changes in the patient's measures regularly in order to inform treatment decisions.
Recovering Quality of Life (ReQoL-10 & ReQoL-20)	A 10- and 20-item measure tapping components of recovering quality of life (Keetharuth et al., 2018).
Reliable and clinically significant improvement	A stringent criterion of improvement that requires a patient's score to show: (1) statistically reliable change; and (2) clinically significant change.
ROAMER	A Roadmap for Mental Health Research in Europe.
Routine outcome measurement	Measurement sampled routinely but not used to adapt the course of therapy.
Routine Outcome Monitoring (ROM)	The most generic term used for referring to ROM that includes feedback.
Routine outcome monitoring feedback	A term used to refer to ROM which emphasizes the inclusion of feedback (only because it is not referred to explicitly in the term ROM).

Scaffolding	A metaphor for referring to the process with a patient of building new knowledge on top of currently available knowledge, thereby providing a direct connection in their mind with existing knowledge.
Sensitivity to change	Psychometric evidence that an outcome measure is sensitive to showing change over time in response to changes made by a patient.
Session Rating Scale (SRS)	A four-item visual analogue measure of alliance within a therapy session (Duncan et al., 2003). It measures relationship, goals, approach and overall experience.
Signal cases	These are patients who are 'not-on-track' as indicated by their outcome measures, and by comparison to clinical norms derived from other patients.
Social Phobia Inventory (SPIN)	A 17-item self-report outcome measure assessing social anxiety. Permission to use the SPIN needs to be obtained from the developer.
Standardized measures	This term refers to any outcome measure that is administered, scored and interpreted in a standard (agreed) way such that data sampled in differing situations can be compared fairly.
Stepped wedge design	A research design in which the potential sample are divided into, for example, four groups and the intervention is introduced to the first subsample and not to the others; (who act as a control). Then it is also introduced to the second subsample so that there are then two subsamples with the intervention compared with the remaining ones (controls). This carries on until all subsamples are assigned the intervention, which can be evaluated against the controls. It is a popular design when rolling out a new intervention and makes it more manageable with the advantage that lessons can be learned along the way so that the intervention can be adjusted to benefit subsequent subsamples.
Substance Abuse and Mental Health Services Administration (SAMHSA)	The major US agency within the Department of Health and Human Services leading efforts to advance the behavioural health of the nation.

Sudden gain/sudden loss	A phenomenon in which patients make dramatic gains (improvement), or losses (deterioration), from one session to another as measured by weekly-administered outcome measures.
Symptom Checklist-Revised-90-R (SCL-R-90)	A 90-item self-report outcome measure that purportedly measures 9 subscales (Derogatis, 1975). It is a proprietary measure.
Treatment Outcome Package (TOP)	This is a treatment package, the main part of which is the TOP-Clinical Scale comprising a 58-item measure tapping 12 symptom and functioning domains of a person's current life (Kraus & Castonguay, 2010). TOP is a proprietary, yet royalty-free tool. It is centrally scored and reported by Outcome Referrals.
Universal Declaration of Ethical Principles for Psychologists	A commitment by the psychology community to uphold ethical principles based on commonly held human values.
Work and Social Adjustment Scale (WSAS)	A five-item measure of functioning (Mundt et al., 2002).

References

Aas, I. H. (2011). Guidelines for rating global assessment of functioning (GAF). *Annals of General Psychiatry, 10*(1), 1–11.

Achenbach, T. M. (1991). *Manual for the Child Behavior Checklist/4-18 and 1991 profile*. Department of Psychiatry, University of Vermont.

Achenbach, T. M., McConaughy, S. H., Ivanova, M. Y., & Rescorla, L. A. (2011). *Manual for the ASEBA brief problem monitor (BPM)*. ASEBA.

Ægisdóttir, S., White, M. J., Spengler, P. M., Maugherman, A. S., Anderson, L. A., Cook, R. S., ... & Rush, J. D. (2006). The meta-analysis of clinical judgment project: Fifty-six years of accumulated research on clinical versus statistical prediction. *The Counseling Psychologist, 34*(3), 341–382.

Alfonsson, S., Parling, T., Spännargård, Å., Andersson, G., & Lundgren, T. (2018). The effects of clinical supervision on supervisees and patients in cognitive behavioral therapy: A systematic review. *Cognitive Behaviour Therapy, 47*(3), 206–228.

American Psychological Association (2015). Guidelines for clinical supervision in health service psychology. *American Psychologist, 70*, 33–46.

American Psychological Association, Presidential Task Force of Evidence-Based Practice (2006). Evidence-based practice in psychology. *American Psychologist, 61*(4), 271–285. doi:10.1037/0003-066X.61.4.271

Anderson, T., McClintock, A. S., Himawan, L., Song, X., & Patterson, C. L. (2016). A prospective study of therapist facilitative interpersonal skills as a predictor of treatment outcome. *Journal of Consulting and Clinical Psychology, 84*(1), 57.

Barkham, M., Bewick, B., Mullin, T., Gilbody, S., Connell, J., Cahill, J., Mellor-Clark, J., Richards, D., Unsworth, G., & Evans, C. (2013). The CORE-10: A short measure of psychological distress for routine use in the psychological therapies. *Counselling and Psychotherapy Research, 13*(1), 3–13.

Barkham, M., & Lambert, M. J. (2021). The efficacy and effectiveness of the psychological therapies. In M. Barkham, W. Lutz & L. G. Castonguay (Eds.), *Bergin and Garfield's handbook of psychotherapy and behavior change* (7th ed. pp. 135–189). Wiley.

Barkham, M., Margison, F., Leach, C., Lucock, M., Mellor-Clark, J., Evans, C., Benson, L., Connell, J., Audin, K., & McGrath, G. (2001). Service profiling and outcomes benchmarking using the CORE-OM: Toward practice-based evidence in the psychological therapies. *Journal of Consulting and Clinical Psychology, 69*(2), 184.

Barkham, M., Mellor-Clark, J., & Stiles, W. B. (2015). A CORE approach to progress monitoring and feedback: Enhancing evidence and improving practice. *Psychotherapy, 52*(4), 402.

Barkham, M., Stiles, W. B., Lambert, M. J., & Mellor-Clark, J. (2010). Building a rigorous and relevant knowledge base for the psychological therapies. In M. Barkham, G. E. Hardy, & J. Mellor-Clark (Eds.), *Developing and delivering practice-based evidence: A guide for the psychological therapies* (pp. 21–61). Wiley.

Batterham, P. J., Sunderland, M., Slade, T., Calear, A. L., & Carragher, N. (2018). Assessing distress in the community: Psychometric properties and crosswalk comparison of eight measures of psychological distress. *Psychological Medicine, 48*(8), 1316–1324.

Beard, J. I., & Delgadillo, J. (2019). Early response to psychological therapy as a predictor of depression and anxiety treatment outcomes: A systematic review and meta-analysis. *Depression and Anxiety, 36*(9), 866–878.

Beck, A. (2016). *Transcultural cognitive behavior therapy for anxiety and depression: A practical guide.* Routledge.

Beck, A. T., Steer, R. A., & Brown, G. K. (1996). *Manual for the Beck Depression Inventory-II.* SanPsychological Corporation.

Benish, S. G., Quintana, S., & Wampold, B. E. (2011). Culturally adapted psychotherapy and the legitimacy of myth: A direct-comparison meta-analysis. *Journal of Counseling Psychology, 58*(3), 279.

Bergman, H., Kornør, H., Nikolakopoulou, A., Hanssen-Bauer, K., Soares-Weiser, K., Tollefsen, T. K., & Bjørndal, A. (2018). Client feedback in psychological therapy for children and adolescents with mental health problems. *Cochrane Database of Systematic Reviews, 8*, CD011729. https://doi.org/10.1002/14651858.CD011729.pub2

Bernard, J. M., & Goodyear, R. K. (2014). *Fundamentals of clinical supervision* (5th ed.). Pearson.

Beutler, L. E., Edwards, C., & Someah, K. (2018). Adapting psychotherapy to patient reactance level: A meta-analytic review. *Journal of Clinical Psychology, 74*(11), 1952–1963.

Bewick, B. M., Trusler, K., Mullin, T., Grant, S., & Mothersole, G. (2006). Routine outcome measurement completion rates of the CORE-OM in primary care psychological therapies and counselling. *Counselling and Psychotherapy Research, 6*(1), 33–40.

Bickman, L. (2008). A measurement feedback system (MFS) is necessary to improve mental health outcomes. *Journal of the American Academy of Child and Adolescent Psychiatry, 47*(10), 1114.

Bickman, L., Douglas, S. R., De Andrade, A. R. V., Tomlinson, M., Gleacher, A., Olin, S., & Hoagwood, K. (2016). Implementing a measurement feedback system: A tale of two sites. *Administration and Policy in Mental Health and Mental Health Services Research, 43*(3), 410–425.

Blais, M. A., Sinclair, S. J., Baity, M. R., Worth, J., Weiss, A. P., Ball, L. A., & Herman, J. (2012). Measuring outcomes in adult outpatient psychiatry. *Clinical Psychology & Psychotherapy, 19*(3), 203–213.

Bone, C., Simmonds-Buckley, M., Thwaites, R., Sandford, D., Merzhvynska, M., Rubel, J., Deisenhofer, A. -K., Lutz, W., & Delgadillo, J. (2021). Dynamic prediction of psychological treatment outcomes: development and validation of a prediction model using routinely collected symptom data. *The Lancet Digital Health, 3*(4), e231–e240.

Bordin, E. S. (1983). A working alliance based model of supervision. *The Counseling Psychologist, 11*(1), 35–42.

Boswell, J. F., & Constantino, M. J. (2022). *Deliberate practice in cognitive behavioral therapy.* American Psychological Association.

Boswell, J. F., Kraus, D. R., Miller, S. D., & Lambert, M. J. (2015). Implementing routine outcome monitoring in clinical practice: Benefits, challenges, and solutions. *Psychotherapy Research, 25*(1), 6–19.

Bradley, W. J., & Becker, K. D. (2021). Clinical supervision of mental health services: A systematic review of supervision characteristics and practices associated with formative and restorative outcomes. *The Clinical Supervisor, 40*(1), 88–111.

Brattland, H., Koksvik, J. M., Burkeland, O., Gråwe, R. W., Klöckner, C., Linaker, O. M., Ryum, T., Wampold, B., Lara-Cabrera, M. L., & Iversen, V. C. (2018). The effects of routine outcome monitoring (ROM) on therapy outcomes in the course of an implementation process: A randomized clinical trial. *Journal of Counseling Psychology, 65*(5), 641–652.

Burlingame, G., Cox, J., Wells, G., Latkowski, M., Justice, D., Carter, C., & Lambert, M. (2005). *The administration and scoring manual of the Youth Outcome Questionnaire.* OQ Measures.

Byrne, S. L., Hooke, G. R., Newnham, E. A., & Page, A. C. (2012). The effects of progress monitoring on subsequent readmission to psychiatric care: A six-month follow-up. *Journal of Affective Disorders, 137*(1–3), 113–116.

Casper, E. S. (2007). The theory of planned behavior applied to continuing education for mental health professionals. *Psychiatric Services, 58*(10), 1324–1329.

Chapman, B. P., Talbot, N., Tatman, A. W., & Brition, P. C. (2009). Personality traits and the working alliance in psychotherapy trainees: an organizing role for the five factor model? *Journal of Social and Clinical Psychology, 28*(5).

Clark, D. M. (2018). Realising the mass public benefit of evidence-based psychological therapies: The IAPT program. *Annual Review of Clinical Psychology, 14*, 159.

Clement, P. W. (1996). Evaluation in private practice. *Clinical Psychology: Science and Practice, 3*(2), 146–159.

Codman, E. A. (1918). *A study in hospital efficiency: As demonstrated by the case report of the first five years of a private hospital.* Thomas Todd Co.

Connolly Gibbons, M. B., Kurtz, J. E., Thompson, D. L., Mack, R. A., Lee, J. K., Rothbard, A., & Crits-Christoph, P. (2015). The effectiveness of clinician feedback in the treatment of depression in the community mental health system. *Journal of Consulting and Clinical Psychology, 83*(4), 748–759.

Connor, K. M., Davidson, J. R., Churchill, L. E., Sherwood, A., Weisler, R. H., & Foa, E. (2000). Psychometric properties of the Social Phobia Inventory (SPIN): New self-rating scale. *The British Journal of Psychiatry, 176*(4), 379–386.

Constantino, M. J., Arnkoff, D. B., Glass, C. R., Ametrano, R. M., & Smith, J. Z. (2011). Expectations. *Journal of Clinical Psychology, 67*(2), 184–192.

Crits-Christoph, P., Ring-Kurtz, S., Hamilton, J. L., Lambert, M. J., Gallop, R., McClure, B., Kulaga, A., & Rotrosen, J. (2012). A preliminary study of the effects of individual patient-level feedback in outpatient substance abuse treatment programs. *Journal of Substance Abuse Treatment, 42*(3), 301–309.

Davidsen, A. H., Poulsen, S., Lindschou, J., Winkel, P., Tróndarson, M. F., Waaddegaard, M., & Lau, M. (2017). Feedback in group psychotherapy for eating disorders: A randomized clinical trial. *Journal of Consulting and Clinical Psychology, 85*(5), 484.

De Jong, K. (2016). Deriving implementation strategies for outcome monitoring feedback from theory, research and practice. *Administration and Policy in Mental Health and Mental Health Services Research, 43*(3), 292–296.

De Jong, K., Conijn, J. M., Gallagher, R., Reshetnikova, A. S., Heij, M., & Lutz, M. C. (2021). Using progress feedback to improve outcomes and reduce drop-out, treatment duration, and deterioration: A multilevel meta-analysis. *Clinical Psychology Review, 85*, 102002.

De Jong, K., & DeRubeis, R. J. (2018). Effectiveness of psychotherapy. In J. N. Butcher & J. M. Hooley (Eds.), *APA handbook of psychopathology: Psychopathology: Understanding, assessing, and treating adult mental disorders* (pp. 705–725). American Psychological Association.

De Jong, K., Nugter, A., Spinhoven, P. (in preparation). Comparing therapists' outcome expectancies and outcomes with two types of outcome monitoring feedback. Unpublished manuscript.

De Jong, K., Segaar, J., Ingenhoven, T., van Busschbach, J., & Timman, R. (2018). Adverse effects of outcome monitoring feedback in patients with personality disorders: A randomized controlled trial in day treatment and inpatient settings. *Journal of Personality Disorders, 32*(3), 393–413.

De Jong, K., van Sluis, P., Nugter, M. A., Heiser, W. J., & Spinhoven, P. (2012). Understanding the differential impact of outcome monitoring: Therapist variables that moderate feedback effects in a randomized clinical trial. *Psychotherapy Research, 22*(4), 464–474.

Delgadillo, J., Branson, A., Kellett, S., Myles-Hooton, P., Hardy, G. E., & Shafran, R. (2020). Therapist personality traits as predictors of psychological treatment outcomes. *Psychotherapy Research, 30*(7), 857–870.

Delgadillo, J., de Jong, K., Lucock, M., Lutz, W., Rubel, J., Gilbody, S., Ali, S., Aguirre, E., Appleton, M., Nevin, J., O'Hayon, H., Patel, U., Sainty, A., Spencer, P., & McMillan, D. (2018). Feedback-informed treatment versus usual psychological treatment for depression and anxiety: a multisite, open-label, cluster randomised controlled trial. *The Lancet Psychiatry, 5*(7), 564–572.

Delgadillo, J., McMillan, D., Gilbody, S., de Jong, K., Lucock, M., Lutz, W., Rubel, J., Aguirre, E., & Ali, S. (2021). Cost-effectiveness of feedback-informed psychological treatment: Evidence from the IAPT-FIT trial. *Behaviour Research and Therapy, 142*, 103873.

Delgadillo, J., Moreea, O., & Lutz, W. (2016). Different people respond differently to therapy: A demonstration using patient profiling and risk stratification. *Behaviour Research and Therapy, 79*, 15–22. https://doi.org/10.1016/j.brat.2016.02.003

Delgadillo, J., Overend, K., Lucock, M., Groom, M., Kirby, N., McMillan, D., Gilbody, S., Lutz, W., Rubel, J. A., & de Jong, K. (2017). Improving the efficiency of psychological treatment using outcome feedback technology. *Behaviour Research and Therapy, 99*, 89–97.

Derogatis, L. R. (1975). Brief Symptom Inventory (Baltimore, Clinical Psychometric Research). *Psychopathology, 27*(1–2), 14–18.

Derogatis, L. R., & Cleary, P. A. (1977). Confirmation of the dimensional structure of the SCL-90: A study in construct validation. *Journal of Clinical Psychology, 33*(4), 981–989.

Derogatis, L. R., & Melisaratos, N. (1983). The brief symptom inventory: an introductory report. *Psychological Medicine, 13*(3), 595–605.

Driver, C., Martin, E. (2002). *Supervising psychotherapy*. London: Sage.

Drozd, J. F., & Goldfried, M. R. (1996). A critical evaluation of the state-of-the-art in psychotherapy outcome research. *Psychotherapy: Theory, Research, Practice, Training, 33*(2), 171–180.

Duffy, K. E. M., Simmonds-Buckley, M., Saxon, D., Delgadillo, J., & Barkham, M. (2022). Early response as a prognostic indicator in person-centered experiential therapy for depression. *Journal of Counseling Psychology, 69*(6), 803–811.

Dunning, D., Heath, C., & Suls, J. M. (2004). Flawed self-assessment: Implications for health, education, and the workplace. *Psychological Science in the Public Interest, 5*(3), 69–106.

Duncan, B. L., Miller, S. D., Sparks, J. A., Claud, D. A., Reynolds, L. R., Brown, J., & Johnson, L. D. (2003). The Session Rating Scale: Preliminary psychometric properties of a "working" alliance measure. *Journal of Brief Therapy, 3*(1), 3–12.

Duncan, B. L., & Reese, R. J. (2015). The Partners for Change Outcome Management System (PCOMS) revisiting the client's frame of reference. *Psychotherapy, 52*(4), 391–401.

Elliott, R., Bohart, A. C., Watson, J. C., & Murphy, D. (2018). Therapist empathy and client outcome: An updated meta-analysis. *Psychotherapy, 55*(4), 399.

Ellis, M. V., D'Iuso, N., & Ladany, N. (2008). State of the art in assessment, measurement, and evaluation of clinical supervision. In A. K. Hess, K. D. Hess, & T. A. Hess (Eds.), *Psychotherapy supervision: Theory, research, and practice* (2nd ed., pp. 473–499). Wiley.

Ellis, M. V. & Ladany, N. (1997). Inferences concerning supervisees and clients in clinical supervision: An integrative review. In C.E. Watkins (Ed.) *Handbook of psychotherapy supervision* (pp. 447–507). John Wiley & Sons.

Ellis, M. V., Ladany, N., Krengel, M., & Schult, D. (1996). Clinical supervision research from 1981 to 1993: A methodological critique. *Journal of Counseling Psychology, 43*(1), 35–50.

Emmelkamp, P. M., David, D., Beckers, T., Muris, P., Cuijpers, P., Lutz, W., Andersson, G., Araya, R., Banos Rivera, R. M., Barkham, M., Berking, M., Berger, T., Botella, C., Carlbring, P., Colom, F., Essau, C., Hermans, D., Hofmann, S. G., Knappe, S., Ollendick, T. H.,… & Vervliet, B. (2014). Advancing psychotherapy and evidence-based psychological interventions. *International Journal of Methods in Psychiatric Research, 23*(S1), 58–91.

Ericsson, K. A., Krampe, R. T., & Tesch-Römer, C. (1993). The role of deliberate practice in the acquisition of expert performance. *Psychological Review, 100*(3), 363.

Evans, C., Connell, J., Barkham, M., Margison, F., McGrath, G., Mellor-Clark, J., & Audin, K. (2002). Towards a standardised brief outcome measure: Psychometric properties and utility of the CORE–OM. *The British Journal of Psychiatry, 180*(1), 51–60.

Evans, C., Margison, F., & Barkham, M. (1998). The contribution of reliable and clinically significant change methods to evidence-based mental health. *Evidence-Based Mental Health, 1*(3), 70–72.

Falender, C. A., & Shafranske, E. P. (2004). *Clinical supervision: A competency-based approach.* American Psychological Association.

Falender, C. A., Burnes, T. R., & Ellis, M. V. (2013). Multicultural clinical supervision and benchmarks: Empirical support informing practice and supervisor training. *The Counseling Psychologist, 41*(1), 8–27.

Farber, E. W. (2010). Humanistic–existential psychotherapy competencies and the supervisory process. *Psychotherapy Theory, Research, Practice, Training, 47*(1), 28–34.

Finch, A. E., Lambert, M. J., & Schaalje, B. G. (2001). Psychotherapy quality control: The statistical generation of expected recovery curves for integration into an early warning system. *Clinical Psychology & Psychotherapy: An International Journal of Theory & Practice, 8*(4), 231–242.

Fleming, I., and Steen, L. (2004). *Supervision and clinical psychology: Theory, practice and perspectives.* Brunner Routledge.

Flückiger, C., Del Re, A., Wampold, B., & Horvath, A. (2019). Alliance in adult psychotherapy. In J. Norcross & M. J. Lambert (Eds.), *Psychotherapy relationships that work* (pp. 24–78). Oxford University Press.

Freitas, G. J. (2002). The impact of psychotherapy supervision on client outcome: A critical examination of 2 decades of research. *Psychotherapy: Theory, Research, Practice, Training, 39*(4), 354–367.

Garb, H. N. (2005). Clinical judgment and decision making. *Annual Review of Clinical Psychology, 1*, 67.

Goldberg, S. B., Babins-Wagner, R., Rousmaniere, T., Berzins, S., Hoyt, W. T., Whipple, J. L., Miller, S. D., & Wampold, B. E. (2016b). Creating a climate for therapist improvement: A case study of an agency focused on outcomes and deliberate practice. *Psychotherapy, 53*(3), 367–375.

Goldberg, S. B., Rousmaniere, T., Miller, S. D., Whipple, J., Nielsen, S. L., Hoyt, W. T., & Wampold, B. E. (2016a). Do psychotherapists improve with time and experience? A longitudinal analysis of outcomes in a clinical setting. *Journal of Counseling Psychology, 63*(1), 1–11.

Goldman, R. N., Vaz, A., & Rousmaniere, T. (2021). *Deliberate practice in emotion-focused therapy.* American Psychological Association.

Green, H., Barkham, M., Kellett, S., & Saxon, D. (2014). Therapist effects and IAPT Psychological Wellbeing practitioners (PWPs): A multi-level modelling and mixed methods analysis. *Behaviour Research and Therapy, 63*, 43–54.

Grove, W. M., & Meehl, P. E. (1996). Comparative efficiency of informal (subjective, impressionistic) and formal (mechanical, algorithmic) prediction procedures: The clinical–statistical controversy. *Psychology, Public Policy, and Law, 2*(2), 293–323.

Grove, W. M., Zald, D. H., Lebow, B. S., Snitz, B. E., & Nelson, C. (2000). Clinical versus mechanical prediction: A meta-analysis. *Psychological Assessment, 12*(1), 19–30.

Gyani, A., Shafran, R., Layard, R., & Clark, D. M. (2013). Enhancing recovery rates: Lessons from year one of IAPT. *Behaviour Research and Therapy, 51*(9), 597–606.

Hall, G. C. N., Ibaraki, A. Y., Huang, E. R., Marti, C. N., & Stice, E. (2016). A meta-analysis of cultural adaptations of psychological interventions. *Behavior Therapy, 47*(6), 993–1014.

Hannan, C., Lambert, M. J., Harmon, C., Nielsen, S. L., Smart, D. W., Shimokawa, K., & Sutton, S. W. (2005). A lab test and algorithms for identifying clients at risk for treatment failure. *Journal of Clinical Psychology, 61*(2), 155–163.

Hansen, J. C., & Warner Jr, R. W. (1971). Review of research on practicum supervision. *Counselor Education and Supervision, 10*(3), 261–272.

Harmon, C. S., Hawkins, E. J., Lambert, M. J., Slade, K., & Whipple, J. L. (2005). Improving outcomes for poorly responding clients: The use of clinical support tools and feedback to clients. *Journal of Clinical Psychology, 61*, 175–185.

Harmon, S. C., Lambert, M. J., Smart, D. M., Hawkins, E., Nielsen, S. L., Slade, K., & Lutz, W. (2007). Enhancing outcome for potential treatment failures: Therapist–client feedback and clinical support tools. *Psychotherapy Research, 17*(4), 379–392.

Hatfield, D., McCullough, L., Frantz, S. H., & Krieger, K. (2010). Do we know when our clients get worse? An investigation of therapists' ability to detect negative client change. *Clinical Psychology & Psychotherapy, 17*(1), 25–32.

Hawkins, P., & Shohet, R. (1989). *Supervision in the helping professions*. Open University Press.

Holloway, E. L., & Neufeldt, S. A. (1995). Supervision: Its contributions to treatment efficacy. *Journal of Consulting and Clinical Psychology, 63*, 207–213.

Hovland, R. T., & Moltu, C. (2019). Making way for a clinical feedback system in the narrow space between sessions: Navigating competing demands in complex healthcare settings. *International Journal of Mental Health Systems, 13*(1), 1–11.

Howard, K. I., Kopta, S. M., Krause, M. S., & Orlinsky, D. E. (1986). Dose–response studies in psychotherapy. *Psychotherapy, 41*(2), 159–164.

Howard, K. I., Moras, K., Brill, P. L., Martinovich, Z., & Lutz, W. (1996). Evaluation of psychotherapy: Efficacy, effectiveness, and patient progress. *American Psychologist, 51*(10), 1059–1064.

Inskipp, F., & Proctor, B. (2001). *Becoming a supervisor*. Cascade.

International Union of Psychological Science. (2008). Universal declaration of ethical principles for psychologists. www.iupsys.net/about/governance/universal-declaration-of-ethical-principles-for-psychologists.html

Jacobson, N. S., & Truax, P. (1991). Clinical significance: A statistical approach to defining meaningful change in psychotherapy research. *Journal of Consulting and Clinical Psychology, 59*(1), 12–19.

Jensen-Doss, A., & Hawley, K. M. (2010). Understanding barriers to evidence-based assessment: Clinician attitudes toward standardized assessment tools. *Journal of Clinical Child & Adolescent Psychology, 39*(6), 885–896.

Joint Commission (2011). Comprehensive accreditation manual for behavioral health care. *Oakbrook Terrace, Illinois: Joint Commission Resources.*

Kadera, S. W., Lambert, M. J., & Andrews, A. A. (1996). How much therapy is really enough?: A session-by-session analysis of the psychotherapy dose-effect relationship. *The Journal of Psychotherapy Practice and Research, 5*(2), 132–151.

Karpen, S. C. (2018). The social psychology of biased self-assessment. *American Journal of Pharmaceutical Education, 82*(5).

Kaslow, N. J. (2004). Competencies in professional psychology. *American Psychologist, 59*(8), 774–781.

Kazdin, A. E. (2008). Evidence-based treatment and practice: new opportunities to bridge clinical research and practice, enhance the knowledge base, and improve patient care. *American Psychologist, 63*(3), 146–159.

Keetharuth, A.D., Brazier, J, Connell, J., Bjorner, J.B., Carlton, J., Taylor Buck, E., Ricketts, T., McKendrick, K., Browne, J., Croudace, T., & Barkham, M. on behalf of the ReQoL Scientific Group. (2018). Recovering Quality of Life (ReQoL): a new generic self-reported outcome measure for use with people experiencing mental health difficulties. *British Journal of Psychiatry, 212*(1), 42–49.

Kemmelmeier, M. (2016). Cultural differences in survey responding: Issues and insights in the study of response biases. *International Journal of Psychology, 51*(6), 439–444.

Kendrick, T., El-Gohary, M., Stuart, B., Gilbody, S., Churchill, R., Aiken, L., Bhattacharya, A., Gimson, A., Brütt, A. L., de Jong, K., & Moore, M. (2016). Routine use of patient reported outcome measures (PROMs) for improving treatment of common mental health disorders in adults. *Cochrane Database of Systematic Reviews, 7*(7), CD011119.

Knaup, C., Koesters, M., Schoefer, D., Becker, T., & Puschner, B. (2009). Effect of feedback of treatment outcome in specialist mental healthcare: Meta-analysis. *The British Journal of Psychiatry, 195*(1), 15–22.

Knight, R. P. (1941). Evaluation of the results of psychoanalytic therapy. *American Journal of Psychiatry, 98*(3), 434–446.

Kopta, M., Owen, J., & Budge, S. (2015). Measuring psychotherapy outcomes with the Behavioral Health Measure-20: Efficient and comprehensive. *Psychotherapy, 52*(4), 442–448.

Kraus, D., & Castonguay, L. G. (2010). Treatment Outcome Package (TOP): Development and use in naturalistic settings. In M. Barkham, G. E. Hardy, & J. Mellor-Clark (Eds.), *Developing and delivering practice-based evidence: A guide for the psychological therapies* (pp. 155–174). Wiley.

Kraus, D.R., Seligman, D.A., & Jordan, J.R. (2005). Validation of a behavioral health treatment outcome and assessment tool designed for naturalistic settings: The Treatment Outcome Package. *Journal of Clinical Psychology, 61*(3), 285–314.

Kroenke, K., Spitzer, R. L., & Williams, J. B. (2001). The PHQ-9: validity of a brief depression severity measure. *Journal of General Internal Medicine, 16*(9), 606–613.

Kühne, F., Maas, J., Wiesenthal, S., & Weck, F. (2019). Empirical research in clinical supervision: A systematic review and suggestions for future studies. *BMC Psychology, 7*(1), 1–11.

Ladany, N., Friedlander, M. L., & Nelson, M. L. (2005*). Critical events in psychotherapy supervision: An interpersonal approach.* American Psychological Association.

Lambert, M. J. (1983). Comments on "a case study of the process and outcome of time-limited counselling". *Journal of Counseling Psychology, 30*(1), 22–25.

Lambert, M. J. (2007). Presidential address: What we have learned from a decade of research aimed at improving psychotherapy outcome in routine care. *Psychotherapy Research, 17*(1), 1–14.

Lambert, M. J., Morton, J. J., Hatfield, D. R., Harmon, C., Hamilton, S., Reid, R. C., Shimokawa, K., Christopherson, C., & Burlingame, G. M. (2004). *Administration and scoring manual for the OQ-45.2 (Outcome Questionnaire).* Wilmington, DE: American Professional Credentialing Services LLC.

Lambert, M. J., & Shimokawa, K. (2011). Collecting client feedback. *Psychotherapy, 48*(1), 72–79.

Lambert, M. J., Whipple, J. L., & Kleinstäuber, M. (2018). Collecting and delivering progress feedback: A meta-analysis of routine outcome monitoring. *Psychotherapy, 55*(4), 520–537.

Lambert, M. J., Whipple, J. L., Hawkins, E. J., Vermeersch, D. A., Nielsen, S. L., & Smart, D. W. (2003). Is It Time for Clinicians to Routinely Track Patient Outcome? A Meta-Analysis. *Clinical Psychology: Science and Practice, 10*(3), 288–301.

Lambert, M. J., Whipple, J. L., Smart, D. W., Vermeersch, D. A., Nielsen, S. L., & Hawkins, E. J. (2001). The Effects of providing therapists with feedback on patient progress during psychotherapy: Are outcomes enhanced? *Psychotherapy Research, 11*(1), 49–68.

Lewis, C. C., Boyd, M., Puspitasari, A., Navarro, E., Howard, J., Kassab, H., Hoffman, M., Scott, K., Lyon, A., Douglas, S., Simon, G., ... & Kroenke, K. (2019). Implementing measurement-based care in behavioral health: A review. *JAMA Psychiatry, 76*(3), 324–335.

Liese, B. S., & Beck, J. S. (1997). Cognitive therapy supervision. In C.E. Watkins (Ed.), *Handbook of psychotherapy supervision* (pp. 114–133). Wiley.

Locke, B. D., Buzolitz, J. S., Lei, P. W., Boswell, J. F., McAleavey, A. A., Sevig, T. D., Dowis, J. D., & Hayes, J. A. (2011). Development of the Counseling Center Assessment of Psychological Symptoms-62 (CCAPS-62). *Journal of Counseling Psychology, 58*(1), 97–109.

Lucock, M., Halstead, J., Leach, C., Barkham, M., Tucker, S., Randal, C., Lloyd, J., Khan, W., Catlow, H., Waters, E., & Saxon, D. (2015). A mixed-method investigation of patient monitoring and enhanced feedback in routine practice: Barriers and facilitators. *Psychotherapy Research, 25*(6), 633–646.

Lutz, W., Deisenhofer, A. -K., Rubel, J., Bennemann, B., Giesemann, J., Poster, K., & Schwartz, B. (2022). Prospective evaluation of a clinical decision support system in psychological therapy. *Journal of Consulting and Clinical Psychology, 90*(1), 90–106.

Lutz, W., De Jong, K., Delgadillo, J. & Rubel, J. A. (2021). Measuring, predicting, and tracking change in psychotherapy. In M. Barkham, W. Lutz, & L. G. Castonguay (Eds.), *Bergin and Garfield's handbook of psychotherapy and behavior change* (7th ed., pp. 89–134). Wiley.

Lutz, W., De Jong, K., & Rubel, J. (2015). Patient-focused and feedback research in psychotherapy: Where are we and where do we want to go? *Psychotherapy Research, 25*(6), 625–632.

Lutz, W., Ehrlich, T., Rubel, J., Hallwachs, N., Röttger, M. A., Jorasz, C., Mocanu, S., Vocks, S., Schulte, D., & Tschitsaz-Stucki, A. (2013). The ups and downs of psychotherapy: Sudden gains and sudden losses identified with session reports. *Psychotherapy Research, 23*(1), 14–24.

Lutz, W., Hofmann, S. G., Rubel, J., Boswell, J. F., Shear, M. K., Gorman, J. M., ... & Barlow, D. H. (2014). Patterns of early change and their relationship to outcome and early treatment termination in patients with panic disorder. *Journal of Consulting and Clinical Psychology, 82*(2), 287–297.

Lutz, W., Lambert, M. J., Harmon, S. C., Tschitsaz, A., Schürch, E., & Stulz, N. (2006). The probability of treatment success, failure and duration—what can be learned from empirical data to support decision making in clinical practice? *Clinical Psychology & Psychotherapy, 13*(4), 223–232.

Lutz, W., Rubel, J. A., Schwartz, B., Schilling, V., & Deisenhofer, A. -K. (2019). Towards integrating personalized feedback research into clinical practice: Development of the Trier Treatment Navigator (TTN). *Behaviour Research and Therapy, 120*, 103438.

Lutz, W., Schwartz, B., & Delgadillo, J. (2022). Measurement-based and data-informed psychological therapy. *Annual Review of Clinical Psychology, 18*, 71–98.

Lutz, W., Schwartz, B., Martín Gómez Penedo, J., Boyle, K., & Deisenhofer, A. -K. (2020). Working towards the development and implementation of precision mental health-care: An example. *Administration and Policy in Mental Health and Mental Health Services Research, 47*(5), 856–861.

McAleavey, A. A., & Moltu, C. (2021). Understanding routine outcome monitoring and clinical feedback in context: Introduction to the special section. *Psychotherapy Research, 31*(2), 142–144.

McIntosh, N., Dircks, A., Fitzpatrick, J., & Shuman, C. (2006). Games in clinical genetic counseling supervision. *Journal of Genetic Counseling, 15*(4), 225–243.

McClintock, A. S., Perlman, M. R., McCarrick, S. M., Anderson, T., & Himawan, L. (2017). Enhancing psychotherapy process with common factors feedback: A randomized, clinical trial. *Journal of Counseling Psychology, 64*(3), 247–260.

Mcguire-Snieckus, R., Mccabe, R., & Priebe, S. (2003). Patient, client or service user? A survey of patient preferences of dress and address of six mental health professions. *Psychiatric Bulletin, 27*(8), 305–308.

Mellor-Clark, J., Cross, S., Macdonald, J., & Skjulsvik, T. (2016). Leading horses to water: Lessons from a decade of helping psychological therapy services use routine outcome measurement to improve practice. *Administration and Policy in Mental Health and Mental Health Services Research, 43*(3), 279–285.

Miller, S. D., Duncan, B. L., Brown, J., Sparks, J. A., & Claud, D. A. (2003). The outcome rating scale: A preliminary study of the reliability, validity, and feasibility of a brief visual analog measure. *Journal of Brief Therapy, 2*(2), 91–100.

Miller, S. D., Duncan, B. L., Sorrell, R., & Brown, G. S. (2005). The partners for change outcome management system. *Journal of Clinical Psychology, 61*(2), 199–208.

Miller, S. D., Hubble, M. A., & Chow, D. (2020). *Better results: Using deliberate practice to improve therapeutic effectiveness.* American Psychological Association.

Milne, D. L. (2009). *Evidence-based clinical supervision: Principles and practice.* John Wiley & Sons.

Milne, D. L. (2014). Beyond the 'acid test': A conceptual review and reformulation of outcome evaluation in clinical supervision. *American Journal of Psychotherapy, 68*(2), 213–230.

Milne, D., & Gracie, J. (2001). The role of the supervisee: 20 ways to facilitate clinical supervision. *Clinical Psychology Forum, 5*, 13–15.

Milne, D., & James, I. (2000). A systematic review of effective cognitive-behavioural supervision. *British Journal of Clinical Psychology, 39*(2), 111–127.

Milne, D. L., Leck, C., & Choudhri, N. Z. (2009). Collusion in clinical supervision: Review and case study in self-reflection. *The Cognitive Behaviour Therapist, 2*(2), 106–114.

Milne, D. L., Leck, C., James, I., Wilson, M., Procter, R., Ramm, L., & Weetman, J. (2012). High fidelity in clinical supervision research. In I. Fleming & L. Steen (Eds.), *Supervision and clinical psychology: Theory, practice and perspectives* (2nd ed., pp. 142–158). Routledge.

Milne, D. L., Sheikh, A. I., Pattison, S., & Wilkinson, A. (2011). Evidence-based training for clinical supervisors: A systematic review of 11 controlled studies. *The Clinical Supervisor, 30*(1), 53–71.

Moltu, C., McAleavey, A. A., Helleseth, M. M., Møller, G. H., & Norberg, S. S. (2021). How therapists and patients need to develop a clinical feedback system after 18 months of use in a practice-research network: a qualitative study. *International Journal of Mental Health Systems, 15*, 43.

Mundt, J. C., Marks, I. M., Shear, M. K., & Greist, J. M. (2002). The Work and Social Adjustment Scale: A simple measure of impairment in functioning. *The British Journal of Psychiatry, 180*(5), 461–464.

National Collaborating Centre for Mental Health. (2018). The Improving Access to Psychological Therapies Manual. www.england.nhs.uk/wp-content/uploads/2018/06/the-iapt-manual.pdf

National Institute for Health and Care Excellence (NICE). (2011). *Common mental health problems: identification and pathways to care.* National Collaborating Centre for Mental Health.

Nietzel, M. T., Russell, R. L., Hemmings, K. A., & Gretter, M. L. (1987). Clinical significance of psychotherapy for unipolar depression: A meta-analytic approach to social comparison. *Journal of Consulting and Clinical Psychology, 55*(2), 156–161.

Nilsen, P. (2020). Making sense of implementation theories, models, and frameworks. In B. Albers, A. Shlonsky, & R. Mildon (Eds.), *Implementation Science* 3.0 (pp. 53–79). Springer.

Ng, M. Y., Schleider, J. L., Horn, R. L., & Weisz, J. R. (2021). Psychotherapy for children and adolescents: From efficacy to effectiveness, scaling, and personalizing. In M. Barkham, W. Lutz, & L. G. Castonguay (Eds.), *Bergin and Garfield's handbook of psychotherapy and behavior change: 50th anniversary edition* (pp. 625–670). John Wiley & Sons, Inc.

Norcross, J. C., & Lambert, M. J. (2018). Psychotherapy relationships that work III. *Psychotherapy, 55*(4), 303–315.

Nordberg, S. S., McAleavey, A. A., Duszak, E., Locke, B. D., Hayes, J. A., & Castonguay, L. G. (2018). The counseling center assessment of psychological symptoms distress index: A pragmatic exploration of general factors to enhance a multidimensional scale. *Counselling Psychology Quarterly, 31*(1), 25–41.

Østergård, O. K., Randa, H., & Hougaard, E. (2020). The effect of using the Partners for Change Outcome Management System as feedback tool in psychotherapy: A systematic review and meta-analysis. *Psychotherapy Research, 30*(2), 195–212.

Page, S., & Wosket, V. (2001). *Supervising the counsellor: A cyclical model* (2nd ed.). Brunner-Routledge.

Patel, N. (2013). Difference and power in supervision: The case of culture and racism. In I. Fleming & L. Steen (Eds.), *Supervision and clinical psychology: Theory, practice and perspectives* (2nd ed., pp. 112–133). Routledge.

Pejtersen, J. H., Viinholt, B. C. A., & Hansen, H. (2020). Feedback-informed treatment: A systematic review and meta-analysis of the partners for change outcome management system. *Journal of Counseling Psychology, 67*(6), 723–735.

Perunovic, M., & Holmes, J. G. (2008). Automatic accommodation: The role of personality. *Personal Relationships, 15*, 57–70.

Power, N., Noble, L., Simmonds-Buckley, M., Kellett, S., Stockton, C., Firth, N., & Delgadillo, J. (2022). Associations between treatment adherence-competence-integrity (ACI) and adult psychotherapy outcomes: A systematic review and meta-analysis. *Journal of Consulting and Clinical Psychology, 90*(5), 427–445.

Probst, T., Kleinstäuber, M., Lambert, M. J., Tritt, K., Pieh, C., Loew, T.H., ... Delgadillo, J. (2020). Why are some cases not on track? An item analysis of assessment for signal cases during inpatient psychotherapy. *Clinical Psychology & Psychotherapy, 27*(4), 559–566.

Probst, T., Lambert, M. J., Loew, T. H., Dahlbender, R. W., Göllner, R., & Tritt, K. (2013). Feedback on patient progress and clinical support tools for therapists: Improved outcome for patients at risk of treatment failure in psychosomatic in-patient therapy under the conditions of routine practice. *Journal of Psychosomatic Research, 75*(3), 255–261.

Probst, T., Lambert, M. J., Loew, T. H., Dahlbender, R. W., & Tritt, K. (2015). Extreme deviations from expected recovery curves and their associations with therapeutic alliance, social support, motivation, and life events in psychosomatic in-patient therapy. *Psychotherapy Research, 25*(6), 714–723.

Prochaska, J. O., & DiClemente, C. C. (1983). Stages and processes of self-change of smoking: Toward an integrative model of change. *Journal of Consulting and Clinical Psychology, 51*(3), 390–395.

Proctor, B. (2000). *Group supervision: A guide to creative practice.* Sage.

Rainer, J. P. (1996). Introduction to the special issue on psychotherapy outcomes [Editorial]. *Psychotherapy: Theory, Research, Practice, Training, 33*(2), 159.

Reese, R. J., Toland, M. D., & Hopkins, N. B. (2011). Replicating and extending the good-enough level model of change: Considering session frequency. *Psychotherapy Research, 21*(5), 608–619.

Reiser, R. P., & Milne, D. L. (2014). A systematic review and reformulation of outcome evaluation in clinical supervision: Applying the fidelity framework. *Training and Education in Professional Psychology, 8*(3), 149–157.

Roth, A. D., & Pilling, S. (2008). *A competence framework for the supervision of psychological therapies.* Research Department of Clinical, Educational and Health Psychology, University College London.

Rousmaniere, T. G., Swift, J. K., Babins-Wagner, R., Whipple, J. L., & Berzins. S. (2016). Supervisor variance in psychotherapy outcome in routine practice. *Psychotherapy Research, 26*(2), 196–205.

Scaife, J. (2008). *Supervision in clinical practice; A practitioner's guide* (2nd ed.). Routledge.

Schiepek, G. K., Stöger-Schmidinger, B., Aichhorn, W., Schöller, H., & Aas, B. (2016). Systemic case formulation, individualized process monitoring, and state dynamics in a case of dissociative identity disorder. *Frontiers in Psychology, 7*, 1545.

Schilling, V. N. L. S., Zimmermann, D., Rubel, J. A., Boyle, K. S., & Lutz, W. (2021). Why do patients go off track? Examining potential influencing factors for being at risk of psychotherapy treatment failure. *Quality of Life Research, 30*(11), 3287–3298.

Scott, K., & Lewis, C. C. (2015). Using measurement-based care to enhance any treatment. *Cognitive and Behavioral Practice, 22*(1), 49–59.

Shalom, J. G., & Aderka, I. M. (2020). A meta-analysis of sudden gains in psychotherapy: Outcome and moderators. *Clinical Psychology Review, 76*, 101827.

Shimokawa, K., Lambert, M. J., & Smart, D. W. (2010). Enhancing treatment outcome of patients at risk of treatment failure: Meta-analytic and mega-analytic review of a psychotherapy quality assurance system. *Journal of Consulting and Clinical Psychology, 78*, 298–311.

Simmons, P., Hawley, C., Gale, T., & Sivakumaran, T. (2010). Service user, patient, client, user or survivor: Describing recipients of mental health services. *The Psychiatrist, 34*(1), 20–23.

Simon, W., Lambert, M. J., Harris, M. W., Busath, G., & Vazquez, A. (2012). Providing patient progress information and clinical support tools to therapists: Effects on patients at risk of treatment failure. *Psychotherapy Research, 22*(6), 638–647.

Simpson-Southward, C., Waller, G., & Hardy, G. E. (2017). How do we know what makes for "best practice" in clinical supervision for psychological therapists? A content analysis of supervisory models and approaches. *Clinical Psychology & Psychotherapy, 24*(6), 1228–1245.

Stoltenberg, C. D., Bailey, K. C., Cruzan, C. B., Hart, J. T., & Ukuku, U. (2014). The integrative developmental model of supervision. In C. E. Watkins, Jr. & D. L. Milne (Eds.), *The Wiley international handbook of clinical supervision* (pp. 576–597). Wiley-Blackwell.

Stoltenberg, C. D., & Delworth, U. (1987). *Supervising counselors and therapists.* Jossey Bass.

Stulz, N., & Lutz, W. (2007). Multidimensional patterns of change in outpatient psychotherapy: The phase model revisited. *Journal of Clinical Psychology, 63*(9), 817–833.

Tam, H. E., & Ronan, K. (2017). The application of a feedback-informed approach in psychological service with youth: Systematic review and meta-analysis. *Clinical Psychology Review, 55*, 41–55.

Tang, T. Z., & DeRubeis, R. J. (1999). Sudden gains and critical sessions in cognitive-behavioral therapy for depression. *Journal of Consulting and Clinical Psychology, 67*(6), 894–904.

Tsui, M. S., O'Donoghue, K., & Ng, A. K. (2014). Culturally competent and diversity-sensitive clinical supervision. An international perspective. In C. E. Watkins, Jr. & D. L. Milne (Eds.), *The Wiley international handbook of clinical supervision* (pp. 238–254). Wiley.

Tugendrajch, S. K., Sheerin, K. M., Andrews, J. H., Reimers, R., Marriott, B. R., Cho, E., & Hawley, K. M. (2021). What is the evidence for supervision best practices? *The Clinical Supervisor, 40*(1), 68–87.

van Oenen, F. J., Schipper, S., Van, R., Schoevers, R., Visch, I., Peen, J., & Dekker, J. (2016). Feedback-informed treatment in emergency psychiatry; a randomized controlled trial. *BMC Psychiatry, 16*(1), 110.

Vetere, A., & Sheehan, J. (Eds.). (2017). *Supervision of family therapy and systemic practice*. Springer

Wahl, I., Meyer, B., Löwe, B. and Rose, M. (2010). Measurement of patient reported outcomes in psychotherapy research. *Journal of Psychosomatic Research, 68*(6), 676.

Walfish, S., McAlister, B., O'Donnell, P., & Lambert, M. J. (2012). An investigation of self-assessment bias in mental health providers. *Psychological Reports, 110*(2), 639–644.

Wakefield, S., Kellett, S., Simmonds-Buckley, M., Stockton, D., Bradbury, A., & Delgadillo, J. (2021). Improving Access to Psychological Therapies (IAPT) in the United Kingdom: A systematic review and meta-analysis of 10-years of practice-based evidence. *The British Journal of Clinical Psychology, 60*(1), 1–37.

Wampold, B. E. (2015). Routine outcome monitoring: Coming of age—With the usual developmental challenges. *Psychotherapy, 52*(4), 458–462.

Wampold, B. E., & Imel, Z. E. (2015). *The great psychotherapy debate: The evidence for what makes psychotherapy work*. Routledge.

Wampold, B. E., & Owen, J. (2021). Therapist effects: History, methods, magnitude. In M. Barkham, W. Lutz, & L. G. Castonguay (Eds.), *Bergin and Garfield's handbook of psychotherapy and behavior change* (7th ed., pp. 297–326). Wiley.

Watkins Jr, C. E. (2011). Does psychotherapy supervision contribute to patient outcomes? Considering thirty years of research. *The Clinical Supervisor, 30*(2), 235–256.

Watkins Jr, C. E. (2020). What do clinical supervision research reviews tell us? Surveying the last 25 years. *Counselling and Psychotherapy Research, 20*(2), 190–208.

Watkins Jr, C. E., & Milne, D. L. (Eds.). (2014). *The Wiley international handbook of clinical supervision*. Wiley.

Watkins Jr, C. E., Vîşcu, L. I., & Cadariu, I. E. (2021). Psychotherapy supervision research: On roadblocks, remedies, and recommendations. *European Journal of Psychotherapy & Counselling, 23*(1), 8–25.

Wheeler, S., & Richards, K. (2007). The impact of clinical supervision on counsellors and therapists, their practice and their clients. A systematic review of the literature. *Counselling and Psychotherapy Research, 7*(1), 54–65.

Whipple, J., Hoyt, T., Rousmaniere, T., Swift, J., Pedersen, T., & Worthen, V. (2020). Supervisor variance in psychotherapy outcome in routine practice: A replication. *SAGE Open, 10*(1), 2158244019899047.

White, M. M., Lambert, M. J., Ogles, B. M., Mclaughlin, S. B., Bailey, R. J., & Tingey, K. M. (2015). Using the Assessment for Signal Clients as a feedback tool for reducing treatment failure. *Psychotherapy Research, 25*(6), 724–734.

Williams, E. (2021). Understanding common obstacles and solutions to deliver effective psychological treatment. Doctor of Clinical Psychology thesis, University of Sheffield, United Kingdom.

Wilson, H. M., Davies, J. S., & Weatherhead, S. (2016). Trainee therapists' experiences of supervision during training: A meta-synthesis. *Clinical Psychology & Psychotherapy, 23*(4), 340–351.

Wright, C. V., Goodheart, C., Bard, D., Bobbitt, B. L., Butt, Z., Lysell, K., McKay, D., & Stephens, K. (2020). Promoting measurement-based care and quality measure development: The APA mental and behavioral health registry initiative. *Psychological Services, 17*(3), 262–270.

Young, C., Schulthess, P., Szyszkowitx, T., Oudijks, R., & Stabingis, A. (2013). The professional competencies of a European psychotherapist: An EAP project. *International Journal of Psychotherapy, 17*(2), 39–57.

Index

Page numbers in italics are figures; with 't' are tables; with 'n' are notes.